FATTY LIVER DIET

Ultimate Fatty Liver Diet Recipes And Guide

105 Recipes To Help Fight Fatty Liver Disease

SHERRY BRANDON

Healthy Quinoa Breakfast Burrito Dish

Beautiful Morning Avocado Salad

SMOOTHIE RECIPES

Smooth Green Smoothie

Super food Green Smoothie Recipe

Liver Good Almond Chocolate Smoothie Bowl

Papaya, Pineapple And Banana Colada

Lemon Strawberry Smoothie

Colorful Pink Smoothie

Coconut Green Smoothie

Full Medal Smoothie

Healthy Super Juice

Healthy Brain Active Smoothie

Cucumber Soy Shake with Coconut

Tasty Ginger, Honey Lemonade

Healthy Pumpkin Spice Latte

Evergreen Pumpkin Spice Smoothie

Gorgeous Berry, Banana, Yogurt Smoothie

SALAD RECIPES

Kelp Noodles Mixed Veggie salad

Real Deal Fresh Vegetable Salad

Avocado, Cajun Sweet Potato Salad

Liver Treat Chunky Avocado Salsa

Grandma Style Mixed Vegetables

Special Easy Salad

Salad Tangorana

Ageing Resistance Salad

Pumpkin Seeds With Kale And Strawberry Salad

Guacamole Salad Thyroid-Friendly

Mixed Bell Pepper, Avocado And Corn Salad

Super Simple Salad

Liver Rescue Vegetable "Bone" Broth

Super Green soup

Sweet Potato & Kale Chili

SOUP RECIPES

Creamy Soup

Butternut Squash Creamy Soup

Coconut, Pumpkin-Cauli- Soup

Nutritious Green Soup

Vegetable Zucchinis Soup

Ginger Broccoli And Spinach Soup

Creamy Red Lentil And Kale Soup

Liver Healthy Healing Soup

Justified Broccoli-Creamy Avocado Soup

Cauliflower Soup

Friendly Meatless Soup

Best Liver Healing Mushroom Soup

Arugula And Broccoli Liver Detox Soup

Unique Healthy Soup with Kale

Garnished Pear Soup Red

LUNCH RECIPES

Hemp Seeds With Spicy Steamed Greens

Healthy Roasted Brussels Sprouts & Vinaigrette

Easy Veggie Hash

Pleased Stuffy Sweet Potatoes

Hearty Meatless Pie

Creamy Mushroom Omelet

Oven Baked Black Bean Brownies

Liver Pass Fresh Turmeric Rice

Mushrooms Oregano toasted wheat rolls

Special Turkey With Veggie Stuffed Peppers

Spinach Zucchini With Pesto

Papaya- Avocado Salad

Easy Healthy Risotto

Unique Quinoa Stuffed Squash

Roasted Cauliflower And Coriander

DINNER RECIPES

Quick Greens And Beans

Seasoned Cauliflower Rice With Beans

Liver Friendly Pesto Pasta Salad

Simple Steps Quinoa Salad

Simple Steps Dinner Dish

Dinner Style Smoothie Bowl

Spaghetti Squash Stuffed With Vegetable

Chickpea Chili Quinoa with Sweet Potato

Healthy Liver Friendly Chilli Chicken

Delicious Turkey Meatloaf

Amazing Lime Rice With Garlic Cilantro

Sweet Potato, Mushrooms-Chickpea Cacciatore

Liver Friendly Roasted Broccoli

Mashed parsley Cauliflower Potatoes

Quinoa, white beans Sweet Potato With Carrot

DESSERT AND SNACK

Almond- Cinnamon Porridge, Grain-Free

Smooth Sailing Muffin Crumble

Vegan Pineapple Coconut Whip

No season Apple Pie Chia Parfait

Healing Macadamia Cashew Peanut Butter

Seasoned Green Bean

Cucumber With Tuna Mixture

Banana Garnished Chia Seed Pudding

Collard Greens Coconut vinegar Wrap

Healthy Liver Mashed Avocado Wraps

Healthy Pumpkin Fries

Best Marinated Zucchini Squash

American Spicy Stewed Apples

Granola Oats Bars Dessert

Gifted Plum Muffin Crumble

INTRODUCTION

What is fatty liver?

Fatty liver, and also called "hepatic steatosis" is a situation where fat has been built-up in the liver. It's not strange to have a little measure of fat present in your liver, but having it in excess can result into a health issue. If excess fat is built up in the liver, it hinders the liver from functioning to its full capacity which pose a real health danger.

How The Liver Works In The Body

The liver is the second largest organ in the body and it has variety of function like:

Metabolism of carbohydrates, fats and proteins

Excretion of hormones, bilirubin, cholesterol and drugs

Enzyme activation

It helps to synthesize plasma proteins

It stores glycogen, minerals and vitamins,

Blood purification and detoxification

Production of bile and the excretion

Types of fatty liver disease

Fatty liver is divided into two types: Alcoholic fatty liver disease, also called alcoholic steatohepatitis and (NAFLD) nonalcoholic fatty liver disease.

Nonalcoholic Fatty Liver Disease:

Nonalcoholic Fatty Liver Disease is the most common type of fatty liver disease, though this type of condition is usually not harmful but sometimes people may develop an advanced stage of it, called (NASH) nonalcoholic steatohepatitis. Recently, there have been an increasing rate of nonalcoholic fatty liver disease (NAFLD). While the major cause of NAFLD can be traced down to poor diet. But you're more likely to if you're obese or overweight; high blood pressure, have diabetes, triglycerides and high cholesterol or other liver infections. Patients with suspected or confirmed diagnosis are advice to follow a nutritional recommendations, should consider a switch from the consumption of mainly refined grains to whole grains. Aside eating a healthy diet, there is also a need for an increase in physical activity to promote weight loss.

At an advance stage of fatty liver nonalcoholic fatty liver "steatohepatitis", your liver becomes swollen and can also cause cirrhosis (when you have a scare on your liver that won't heal).
This can open a door to issues like:
Esophageal varices: which is the swelling of veins in the esophagus
Having heart disease
Chance of liver cancer
Drowsiness, Confusion and slurred speech (hepatic encephalopathy)
Liver failure, when your liver finally stops functioning
Ascites: fluid buildup in the abdomen

Alcoholic fatty liver disease:
The alcoholic steatohepatitis, which is an early fatty liver disease stage, people who take alcohol is excess are at high risk of it. Drinking excessively can damage the liver, and this can hinder the liver from perform the function of breaking down fat properly. If your alcohol consumption is not put under check it can lead to higher chance of liver cancer, liver failure, alcoholic hepatitis or cirrhosis.

Who Is At Risk Of Fatty Liver Disease?
People with a higher risk of developing fatty liver diseases are people that are overweight or obese. People with type 2 diabetes also stand a greater risk of fatty liver disease.
Other factors that add to the risk for fatty liver:
High cholesterol
High triglyceride levels
Malnutrition
Absent of good physical activity
Underactive pituitary gland (hypopituitarism)
Pregnancy
Over use of some certain medications, like as acetaminophen (Tylenol)

Metabolic syndrome
Underactive thyroid (hypothyroidism)
Metabolic syndrome
Excessive consumption of alcohol

What Are The Known Symptoms of Fatty Liver

The unfortunate thing about this is most people living with fatty liver disease do not know that they have it. Sadly there is a great danger if left untreated.

There are no specific symptoms for fatty liver disease, but at a point, some people might experience different symptoms like:

Nausea
Abdominal pain
Vomiting
Loss of appetite
Become very tired
Jaundice
Excessive weight loss and nausea.

How to diagnose a Fatty Liver?

Blood tests

Running a blood test may help to discover the risk of fatty liver, if there is an
unusual increase in the liver enzymes during a routine blood test, this can be related
to liver inflammation but does not ascertain a fatty liver disease, although further
analysis should be carried out.

Fibro Scan

Similar to ultra sound, it makes use of sound waves to determine the normal liver tissue, density of the liver and correlating areas of fat.

Liver biopsy
This is still regarded as most effective way to detect the severity of liver disease and also the exact cause. It is done by inserting a needle into the liver to extract a piece of tissue, the tissue is then examined to detect a liver disease. A local anesthetic will be given to reduce the pain.

Ultra sound and other imaging studies, using an ultrasound can help to detect fat in your liver, more so other imaging studies can be done as well, such as MRI or CT scans.
It can be detected by your doctor by inspecting your abdomen for an enlarged liver. Though there are cases where the liver might be inflamed and not being enlarged. It's your duty to explain to your doctor if you ever experience loss of appetite or fatigue, also inform him about medication, supplement and alcohol use.

What Can Be Done To Reverse And Treat Fatty Liver?

One important thing you need to do is change your lifestyle.
You can reverse and treat fatty liver disease by eating a well-balanced diet, removing or reducing fatty foods and foods that have high level of sugar from your diet, eat lots of veggies, and avoid red meats, best to eat lean proteins such as fish, turkey, chicken and soy, whole grains, with good-for-you fats
Sodas, juices and any sweet drink should be eliminated.

You can reverse fatty liver automatically, when the necessary steps is taken to treat obesity, an unhealthy diet, diabetes, and high cholesterol,

Making effort to prevent having a liver disease.

Exercise regularly, it helps you to get rid of excess liver fat. Small workout, brisk walking etc.
Stop drinking alcohol. This might not be easy for some people but it's something you need to work on for your overall health benefit.

Reduce carbs and sugar intake

Be kind to your liver, mindful of your medications, especially the ones that can cause fatty liver.

Foods to Eat

1. Walnuts

Walnuts are high in omega-3 fatty acids which helps to improved liver.

2. Olive oil for weight control

Olive oil has high in omega-3 fatty acids f omega-3 fatty acids which can assist to lower liver enzyme levels, bring down inflammation and improve liver fat levels.

3. Oatmeal

Oatmeal have fiber content that can help weight maintenance, more so the Carbohydrates present in whole grains like oatmeal is a good source of body energy.

4. Milk and other low-fat dairy

Milk and other low-fat dairy may assist to protect the liver from more damage because of the presence of whey protein

5. Fish for inflammation and fat levels

Fish such as trout, tuna, sardines, and salmon, have high level of omega-3 fatty acids which can assist bringing down inflammation and improve liver fat levels.

6. Garlic

Apart from adding flavor to food, it also help reduce fat and body weight in people with fatty liver disease. Research have made known that people that love to drink coffee have lesser risk of liver damage. Caffeine helps to reduce abnormal liver enzymes and risk of liver diseases.

7. Sunflower seeds as antioxidants

Vitamin E are high antioxidant that helps to protect the liver from damage. Sunflower seeds are rich in vitamin E.

8. Tofu to reduce fat buildup

Tofu high in protein and low in fat. Soy protein present tofu, helps lower fat buildup in the liver.

9. Avocado help protect the liver

Fruits like avocados and nuts. Avocados contain chemicals that have the ability to slow liver damage and are also rich in healthy fats.

10. Greens to prevent fat buildup

Eat enough greens, like kale, spinach, Brussels sprouts, and spinach. It help to reduce weight. Spinach is help prevent fat building up in the liver.

11. Fruits Especially citrus fruits, it has essential vitamins that is beneficial for the health and has great potential for fatty liver treatment.

12. Green tea for less fat absorption

Green tea improve liver function and storage in the liver and. Green tea is also beneficial in many ways, aiding with sleep and rom lowering cholesterol.

13 Coffee helps to reduce abnormal liver enzymes

Foods to Avoid

Alcohol a major cause of fatty liver disease.

Salt. Consuming too much salt can cause the body holding on to excess water. It is advice to reduce sodium to 1,400 ml or less per day.

Red meat. Deli meats and Beef are high in saturated fat which is not good for the liver.

Pasta, white bread, rice. White normally translate the flour is highly processed, which is not good for your blood sugar because it can raise the blood level.

Fried foods are high in calories and fat.

Added sugar, such as fruit juices, sodas, cookies and candy. High blood sugar increases the amount of fat buildup in the liver.

BREAKFAST RECIPES

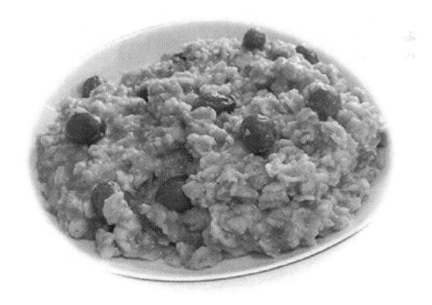

Milky Oatmeal breakfast

Prep: 5 mins
Cook time: 8 hrs
Servings: 4

Ingredients:

1/2 tsp of cinnamon
2 tbsp of brown sugar
1/3 cup of golden raisins
1 cup of steel cut oats
2 cups of skim milk
2 cups of water
1/4 tsp of salt

Preparations:

1. combine the water, cinnamon ,brown sugar, golden raisins, steel cut oats, skim milk, and salt In a 4 quart slow cooker, stir ingredients together gently with a large spoon until they are well combined.
2. Reduce to low heat with the lid on, and cook until the oats are soft and completely cooked, about 7 to 8 hours. Transfer into a serving bowls. Serve with additional milk if you wish.

Mixed Breakfast Salad

Prep time: 10 minutes
Total time: 10 minutes
Servings: 2 servings

Ingredients:

Salad:
2 tablespoons of shredded coconut
½ large mango, thickly slices
2 pineapple, thickly slices
1/3 papaya, thickly slices
Dressing:
(Optional) 1-2 teaspoon of Stevia
1 tsp of lemon zest
2 tsp of lemon juice
½ cup of Greek yogurt

Preparations:
1. Lightly toast the coconut over a medium to low heat in a small pan.
2. Place the fruit slices on a plate
3. Combine dressing ingredients together then drizzle on the fruit slices then top with the lightly toasted coconut and enjoy.
Note: If you want to store for the next day, simply keep the fruit and yogurt separate.

Apple with Almond Milk And Oats

Prep time: 5 mins
Cook time 3 mins
Servings: 2

Ingredients:
1 tablespoon of walnuts chopped
1 1/2 tablespoon of dates, finely chopped
1 cup of readymade almond milk
1/2 cup of quick cooking rolled oats
1/4 tsp of cinnamon powder
1/4 cup of apple, chopped (unpeeled)

Preparations:
1. In a large non-stick pan over on a medium heat, add together the cinnamon powder, dates, almond milk, and oats, cook for 2 to 3 minutes, stirring occasionally.
2. Add the walnuts and apples mix thoroughly. Serve immediately.

Liver Embraced Granola Breakfast

Prep time: 3 mins

Cook time 35-40 mins

Servings: 1-2

Ingredients:

1 cup of dried cranberries, or preferred dried chopped fruit

1/3 cup of apple cider or apple juice

1/3 cup of good honey

1/3 cup of applesauce

1/2 teaspoon of salt

1/4 teaspoon of nutmeg

1/2 teaspoon of cinnamon

3 tbsp of brown sugar

1 cup of shredded coconut

2 tbsp of flax seeds

1/2 cup of hazelnuts, chopped

1/2 cup of almonds, chopped

4 cups of organic rolled oats (it's different from quick cooking oats)

Preparations:

1. Heat up the oven to 300 F. Stir the nutmeg, cinnamon, coconut, flax seeds, brown sugar, nuts, oats and salt together in a large mixing bowl.

2. Whisk the apple juice, honey, and applesauce together in a different bowl.

3. Combine the wet mixture with the dry mixture and stir until you have a well-combined mixture.

4. Lined parchment paper over a large sheet pan and spread the granola onto the pan. 5. Bake in the oven and keep stirring once in 10 minutes, until the mixture turns golden brown and nice, about 30 to 40 minutes.

5. Withdraw from the oven and let granola cool completely, stirring once a bit. Stir in the cranberries.

You can eat Granola plain with some almond milk or with yogurt. Can be stored in a plastic bag or an airtight container and refrigerate for weeks.

Banana Crushed Cold-Busting Oats

Prep time: 5 minutes

Cook time: 15 minutes

Servings: 2

Ingredients:

 1/2 teaspoon of maple syrup

1/2 teaspoon of coconut oil

1/4 teaspoon of ground ginger

1/2 teaspoon of cinnamon

1/4 teaspoon of sea salt

1/4 (40 g) cup of cranberries

 1 fresh or frozen banana

2 (500 ml) cups of water

1(90 g) cup of gluten-free rolled oats

Preparations:

1. Bring water to a boil in a small pot, you can add salt if desired.

2. Reduce heat and add oats then simmer on low.

3. Add maple syrup, coconut oil, ginger, cinnamon, cranberries and banana.

4. Stir briefly to crush the banana into oats until desired constituency is reached.

5. Turn heat off and Cover to sit for 2 minutes. Stir and enjoy!

A Healthy Liver Breakfast

Prep time: 5 minutes
Cook time: 5 minutes
Servings: 1

Ingredients:

Pinch Himalayan or Sea salt
½ sliced peach
3-4 large chopped Brazil nuts
¼ cup of organic grits
1 cup of water

Preparations:

1. Pour water into a pot, bring to a boil and stir in grits, reduce heat to low and cook with the lid on, about 5 minutes, stirring not too often.
2. Remove the grits from heat when its ready, then pour into a bowl.
3. Top with chopped nuts and slices of peach. Season with salt. Enjoy!

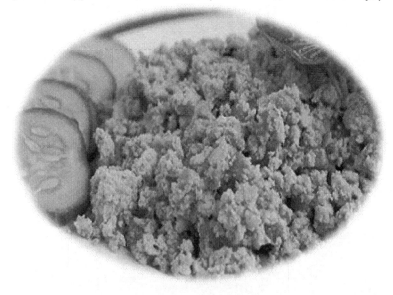

Brief Garlic Hummus

Prep time: 15 mins

Cook time 0 mins

Servings: 1

Ingredients:

1/4 teaspoon of olive oil, for drizzling

1 1/2 tablespoon of olive oil

1/2 tablespoon of garlic, roughly chopped

1 tablespoon of red chili paste

1/4 cup of curds

 2 tbsp of water

Salt to taste

1 cup of white chick peas (soaked and boiled)

Preparations:

1. Add every ingredients together in a mixer and blend till smooth.

2. Add a drizzle of oil and serve chilled.

Liver Embraced Steel Cut Oats with Almond Milk And Strawberries

Prep time: 10 mins

Cook time 8 mins

Servings: 2

Ingredients:

1 tbsp of roasted almond halves

2 tsp of maple syrup

1/4 tsp of vanilla essence

1/2 cup of almond milk

3/4 cup of strawberry cubes

1/2 cup of steel cut oats, soak in water for 8 hours, drain.

Preparations:

1. Measure a cup of water and boil in a non-stick pan, add oats and mix well.

2. Cook with the lid on over medium low heat for 6 minutes, stirring not too often.

3. Pour the mixture to cool into a large bowl.

4. Add the maple syrup, ½ cup of strawberries vanilla essence and almond milk, and stir well.

5. Top with roasted almonds and the reserved ¼ cup of strawberries. Serve right away or store in the fridge.

Simple Yogurt Custard Chia Seed

Prep time: 10 mins
Cook time: 10 mins
Servings: 2 cups

Ingredients:
6 tbsp of chia seeds
1/2 tsp of cinnamon
1/2 tsp of ground sumac
1/4 cup of freshly squeezed orange juice
3/4 cup of coconut milk
1/2 tsp of vanilla extract
1 cup of kefir yogurt or plain live
2 tbsp of honey

Preparations:
1. Combine sumac, cinnamon and chia seeds in a blender and blend just enough to form a coarse powder.

2. Add honey, milk, yogurt, vanilla and orange juice. Blend about four or five times, the consistency of the mixture should resemble a thick soup.

3. Let set about an hour or overnight in the fridge to form a thicker, custard like mix.

Stylish Healthy Oatmeal

Prep time: 10 mins

Cook time 8 mins

Servings: 2

Ingredients:

1 cup of water

1 teaspoon of clover honey

1 teaspoon of pure maple syrup

½ cup of raisins (organic, if possible)

1 teaspoon of ground cinnamon.

½ cup of steel rolled oats

Preparations:

1. Cook Steel rolled oats according to manufacturer directions. You can add salt if you want. Add remaining ingredients and stir thoroughly.

Healthy Liver Friendly Quinoa Bowl

Servings: 2

Ingredients:

4 tablespoon of soaked almonds

2 teaspoon of olive oil

2 cup of cooked broccoli

1 cup of cooked quinoa

Coriander, parsley and Sea salt to Seasoning

Preparations:

1. In a bow, add all the ingredients. Enjoy!

Simple Liver Friendly Chia Seed Pudding

Servings: 2

Ingredients:

1 tablespoon of honey

½ cup of berries

2 cup vanilla almond milk, unsweetened (or coconut milk)

½ cup of chia seeds

Preparations:

1. Mix honey, chia seeds and coconut milk or almond in small glass. Place in the fridge overnight to set.

2. It should be thick by morning and the chia seeds have gelled. Remove and top with berries. Enjoy!

Liver Friendly Seed Muesli And Soaked Almond

Servings: 1

Ingredients:

1 cup of unsweetened almond milk

1 tablespoon of flaxseeds

1 tablespoon of chia seeds

¼ cup of raw pumpkin seeds

¼ cup of raw almonds

Cinnamon and stevia to taste

Preparations:

1. Place all ingredients in a bowl, season with cinnamon and stevia to taste.

2. Allow to soak overnight. Enjoy your tasty breakfast in the morning!

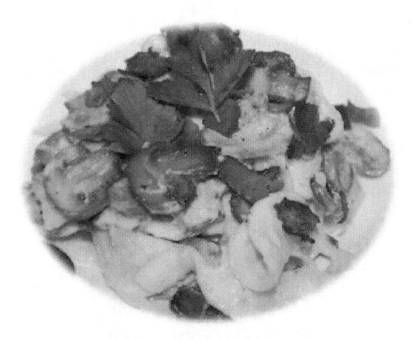

Healthy Quinoa Breakfast Burrito Dish

Prep time: 10 mins
Cook time: 35 mins
Serving: 2

Ingredients:

Handful of chopped cilantro
2 sliced avocados
1 teaspoon cumin
4 minced cloves garlic
2 freshly juiced limes
4 green sliced onions
2 15-oz cans of adzuki beans, rinsed and drained
2 cups of filtered water
1 cup of quinoa

Preparations:

1. Add the water in a pot and cook the quinoa over high heat.
2. Cover and reduce heat to low immediately the water comes to a boil, cook for 15-20 minutes or until quinoa is cooked and water is absorbed.
3. Meanwhile, cook beans on low heat in a small saucepan. Stir cumin, garlic, lime juice, and onions, cook for 10 to 15 minutes.

4. Serve quinoa into different serving bowls, top with cilantro, beans and avocado. Enjoy!

Beautiful Morning Avocado Salad

Servings: 1

Ingredients:

Half a lemon juice

Half a red onion, chopped

2 tomatoes, chopped

One spoon of chili sauce

4 handfuls of baby spinach

A handful of chopped almonds

1 pink chopped grapefruit

1 Avocado, chopped

Half a pack of firm tofu, chopped

2 Tortillas

Preparations:

1. Heat the tortillas in the oven for 8 to 10 minutes.

2. Combine tomatoes, tofu and onions with some chilli sauce in a bowl, place inside the refrigerator to cool.

3. Add the avocado, grapefruit and almonds. Mix everything together and place into the bowl.

4. Top with a Squeeze of fresh lemon juice!

SMOOTHIE RECIPES

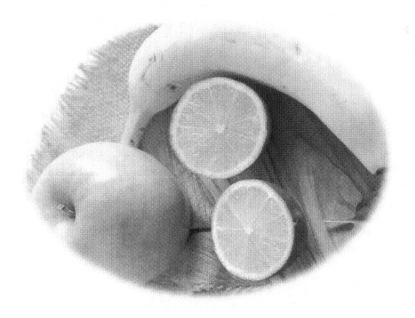

I prefer to use a Vita-mix blender for my smoothie

Smooth Green Smoothie

Prep: 5 mins

Servings: 2

Ingredients:

2 cups of Filtered water

(Optional) 1 tsp of grated ginger

1 Fuji apple, cut in chunks

(Optional) 1 small banana broken into 1" pieces

1 peeled organic or Meyer lemon, sliced into 1" chunks

4 (about 2 ½ cups) chopped kale leaves, without stems

6 (about 1 cup) chopped dandelion greens

Preparations:

Combine all ingredients in a blender and blend for 1-2 minutes until you have smooth mixture. You can add more water as desired.

Super food Green Smoothie Recipe

Prep: 5 mins

Servings: 2

Ingredients:

1 cup of fresh spinach

1/4 cup of soy or almond milk

1/2 cup of fresh blueberries

4 cubes of ice

1 banana

Optional: touch of agave nectar

Preparations:

Combine all ingredients in a blender and blend for 1-2 minutes until you have smooth mixture.

Liver Good Almond Chocolate Smoothie Bowl

Prep time: 10 minutes

Servings: 1

Ingredients:

1 scoop protein powder (Optional)

1 date or Stevia to taste

½ cup of almond milk

1/2 teaspoon of vanilla extract

1 Tablespoon of cacao powder

2 Tablespoon of almond butter

1 handful of spinach

½ cup of blueberries

1 frozen banana (Green banana will do just fine)

Toppings: cacao nibs, chia seeds, shredded coconut, chopped nuts, strawberries or blueberries

Preparations:

1. Combine every ingredients in a blender and blend for 1-2 minutes until you have smooth mixture.

2. Transfer mixture into a bowl and add your favorite toppings.

Papaya, Pineapple And Banana Colada

Prep time: 10 minutes

Servings: 1

Ingredients:

2 teaspoon of chia seeds

1 Tablespoon of shredded coconut

½ cup of coconut milk

½ cup of ice

¼ fresh papaya, chopped

(Optional) 1 frozen banana

1/8 of frozen or fresh pineapple, chopped

Preparations:

Combine every ingredients in a blender and blend for 1-2 minutes until you have smooth mixture. Enjoy!

Lemon Strawberry Smoothie

Prep time: 5 minutes
Servings: 1

Ingredients:

8-10 oz unsweetened almond or hemp milk
1 scoop of plant based protein (pea protein, hemp or sprouted rice)
Dash of cinnamon
1 Tablespoon of avocado oil or 1/3 avocado
2 handfuls of romaine lettuce
½ lemon (peel on)
¼ banana
6 strawberries, tops removed

Preparations:

Combine every ingredients in a blender and blend until you have smooth mixture. Enjoy!

Colorful Pink Smoothie

Prep time: 5 minutes
Servings: 1

Ingredients:

½ cup of ice
Dash of turmeric
1 teaspoon of vanilla extract
1 Tablespoon of goji berries
3/4 cup of frozen raspberries
8-10 ounces of almond or hemp milk
2 Tablespoon of cashew butter

Preparations:

Combine every ingredients in a blender and blend until you have smooth mixture. Enjoy!

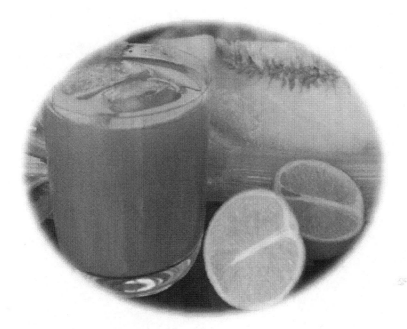

Coconut Green Smoothie

Prep time: 5 minutes

Servings: 1

Ingredients:

8-10 ounces of hemp milk

2 handfuls of spinach

Dash dried turmeric

1 Tablespoon of spirulina or chlorella (blue-green algae)

2 Tablespoon of coconut flakes

1/3 avocado

1 banana

Preparations:

Combine every ingredients in a blender and blend until you have smooth mixture. Enjoy!

Full Medal Smoothie

Prep time: 5 minutes

Servings: 1

Ingredients:

1 handful of mixed greens/arugula

½ cup berries

½ banana

1 scoop plant-based protein

1 teaspoon of almond butter

½ avocado

Preparations:

Combine every ingredients in a blender and blend until you have smooth mixture. Enjoy!

Healthy Super Juice

Prep time: 10 minutes

Servings: 1

Ingredients:

5 stalks of celery

Half lime, peeled

Half bunch of parsley

5 cups of spinach

1 cucumber

Preparations:

Juice all ingredients and enjoy!

Healthy Brain Active Smoothie

Prep time: 5 minutes

Servings: 1 serving

Ingredients:

1 scoop plant based protein (optional)

8 ounces of hemp milk

Dash of cinnamon

Dash of turmeric

2 tablespoon of cacao nibs (best use raw)

2 handfuls of kale

5 strawberries, tops removed

Preparations:

Combine every ingredients in a blender and blend until you have smooth mixture. Enjoy!

Cucumber Soy Shake with Coconut

Serving: 1

Ingredients:

7 cubes of ice

1 teaspoon of organic vanilla

 2 small shredded cucumbers

50ml fresh unsweetened coconut milk, 500ml

Fresh unsweetened soy milk, 500ml

Preparations:

1. Combine all the ingredients in a blender blend until smooth in less 1 minute.

Tasty Ginger, Honey Lemonade

Prep time: 2 mins

Cook time 13 mins

Servings: 8

Ingredients:

2 medium sprigs of fresh rosemary

Ice cubes

1 large sprig of fresh rosemary for garnish, if desired

Lemon slices for garnish, if desired

Juice of 4 lemons

4 large strips of lemon peel

2 tbsp of fresh ginger root, grated

1/3 cup of honey

Preparations:

1. Combine 2 sprigs rosemary, lemon peel, ginger, honey and add 2 cups of water in a small pot.

2. Bring to a boil, then simmer on low heat, for 10 minutes, stirring frequently.

3. Let cool about 15 minutes then strain mixture into large pitcher. Discard the rosemary and ginger.

4. Add lemon juice and six cups of cold water to pitcher, mix to combine.

5. To serve, pour over ice with lemon slice and little piece of fresh rosemary as garnish if desired.

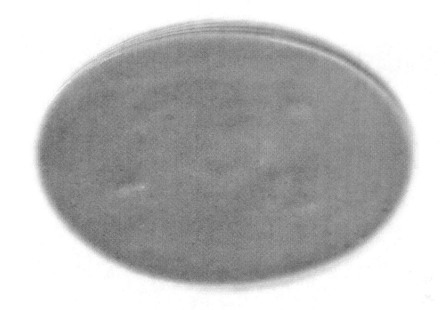

Healthy Pumpkin Spice Latte

Prep time: 5 mins

Cook time 5 mins

Servings: 1

Ingredients:

Pinch of cinnamon

8 ounces of fresh-brewed coffee

2-3 drops of liquid stevia

1/2 tsp of vanilla, alcohol-free

1 tsp of pumpkin pie spice

3 tbsp of pumpkin puree

1/2 cup of vanilla almond milk, unsweetened

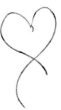

Preparations:

1. Combine pumpkin and almond milk together in a saucepan, and cook over medium heat until hot (not boiling) or place in the microwave for 30 to 45 seconds.

2. Stir in spices, vanilla, and sweetener.

3. Transfer the mix to a blender and blend or until foamy, about 30 seconds.

4. Add the milk mixture into coffee, and top with cinnamon.

Evergreen Pumpkin Spice Smoothie

Prep time: 4 mins

Cook time 2 mins

Servings: 1

Ingredients:

1 handful of ice cubes

1 scoop of Ultra Nourish

Pinch of allspice

Pinch of ground cloves

Pinch of ground nutmeg

¼ teaspoon of ground ginger

¼ teaspoon of ground cinnamon

l tablespoon honey

½ banana

½ cup of canned pumpkin

 1 cup sweetened, vanilla almond milk

Preparations:

1. Combine all the ingredient in a blender and blend to have a smooth mixture.

2. Adjust spice and sweetness to taste, serve and enjoy!

Gorgeous Berry, Banana, Yogurt Smoothie

Prep time: 2 mins

Cook time 5 mins

Servings: 1

Ingredients:

1 scoop of Ultra Nourish

1 cup of unsweetened juice of your choice

1 cup of ice

1 (5 ounces) container of Greek yogurt

1/4 cup of blueberries

Several strawberries, halved

1 banana, cut into small sizes

Preparations:

1. Combine all the ingredient in a blender and blend to have a smooth mixture. Enjoy!

SALAD RECIPES

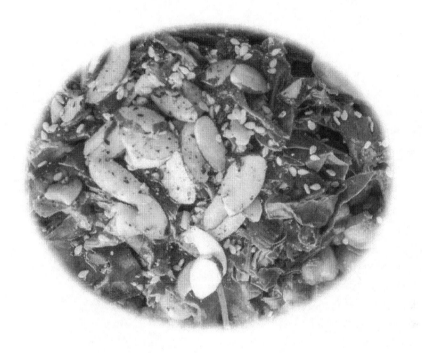

Kelp Noodles Mixed Veggie salad

Prep: 15 mins

Servings: 1

Ingredients:

1 bunch of cilantro (coriander), chopped

1 red onion, thinly sliced

1 cucumber, julienned

1 large zucchini, julienned

1 large carrot, julienned

1 packet of kelp noodles, soak for 15 minute and drain

¼ cup of black sesame seeds

¼ cup of sesame seeds

¾ cup of peanuts

Dressing:

(Optional) 1-2 chopped fresh chili

½ inch grated fresh ginger

1 crushed garlic clove

2 tablespoon of lemon juice

1 tablespoon of apple cider vinegar

3 tablespoon of olive oil

1 tablespoon of sesame oil

2 tablespoon of tahini

3 tablespoon of tamari

Preparations:

1. Toast peanuts and sesame seeds lightly in a pan stirring frequently.

2. Combine all the salad ingredients in a large bowl.

3. Combine all dressing ingredients in a blender and blend for 1-2 minutes until you have smooth mixture.

4. Add dressing to the salad and serve immediately.

Real Deal Fresh Vegetable Salad

Prep time: 10 mins

Cook time: 3 mins

Servings: 1

Ingredients:

1 head romaine lettuce

2 chopped tomatoes

2 shredded carrots

1 diced red bell pepper

1 diced green bell pepper

1 diced small cucumber

1 thinly sliced red onion

Alkalizing Citrus Salad Dressing

Preparations:

1. Combine salad ingredients into a bowl and stir together. Pour the dressing over the salad. Enjoy

Avocado, Cajun Sweet Potato Salad

Servings 4-6

Ingredients:

Lime wedges to serve

2 halved avocados, sliced thick

4 cups of leafy greens

1 crushed clove of garlic

½ cup of pepitas

Cracker pepper to taste

Salt to taste

1 Tablespoon of Cajun spice (¼ chile flakes, 1/2tsp paprika, 1/2 tsp cumin)

1 Tablespoon of melted coconut oil

2 (500g) sweet potatoes

Preparations:

1. Heat up the oven to 350°F.

2. Wash the sweet potato thoroughly (I prefer to have the skin on), slice into ¼ inch discs thick.

3. Mix together the chile flakes, paprika, cumin, garlic, coconut oil, salt and pepper in a bowl. Stir the mixture into the sweet potato.

4. Place in the preheated oven and bake for 15 to 20 minutes until cooked through.

5. Toast pepitas about 5 minutes.

6. Place the greens and other salad ingredients in a bowl, drizzle with your salad dressing and serve with wedges. Enjoy!

Liver Treat Chunky Avocado Salsa

Prep time: 10 mins

Cook time 0 mins

Servings: 2

Ingredients:

½ finely diced spring onion

1 tbsp of avocado or macadamia nut oil

2 tbsp of lime juice

2 tbsp of chopped cilantro leaves

1 large diced ripe tomato

1 large diced avocado

Salt and pepper

Preparations:

1. Add every ingredients together in a bowl and carefully toss. Serve right away.

Grandma Style Mixed Vegetables

Prep time: 10 mins

Cook time 1 hour 20 mins

Servings: 6

Ingredients:

2 tbsp of finely chopped flat-leaf parsley

1 tbsp of dried oregano

1 cup water

1 1/4 cups of tomato passata or puree

5 sliced into rounds small zucchini

12 cherry tomatoes

6 thinly sliced medium tomatoes

1 1/2 lbs (about 4 medium) potatoes cut into 1/2 inch cube

3 sliced garlic cloves

1 thinly sliced large onion

1 large eggplant, sliced lengthwise and cut into half round thick slices

 Salt and fresh ground pepper

1/2 cup of extra-virgin olive oil, plus more if needed

Preparations:

1. Heat up the oven to 425 F.

2. Pour 2 tablespoons of olive oil in a saucepan, heat over medium heat, cook eggplant in batches, about 5–7 minutes and add more oil if needed until the eggplants are golden and softened; Set aside in a bowl.

3. Add garlic and onion to the pan, sauté until softened about 5 minutes. Set aside in the bowl containing the eggplants.

4. Add 1 cup water, passata, zucchini, tomatoes and potato to the bowl. Sprinkle with parsley and oregano and season with ground black pepper and salt. Mix very well to combine, then transfer to a broad ovenproof dish. Drizzle with oil.

5. Place in the preheated oven and bake for 30 minutes.

6. Reduce oven heat to 400 F and bake for 20–30 minutes extra, or until the vegetables are tender and top is brown. Let cool a bit before serving.

Special Easy Salad

Prep time: 15 mins

Cook time 5 mins

Servings: 4

Ingredients:

2 teaspoon of olive oil of high quality

White vinegar

½ pound of green beans cut in 1 inch segments

1 bag of steamed edamame beans,

1 8-12 oz. can of beets

6 large organic carrots, cubed

3 corn on the cobs, corn cut off

Black pepper

Preparations:

1. While wrapped the corn with a damp towel, place microwave for 5 minutes.
2. Steam every ingredients (reserving corn and beets) in large steamer in this other, carrots, green beans, and edamame beans on the top layer.
3. Mix beets together with the cooked ingredients.
4. Blend slightly with a few dashes of black pepper, white vinegar and olive oil.

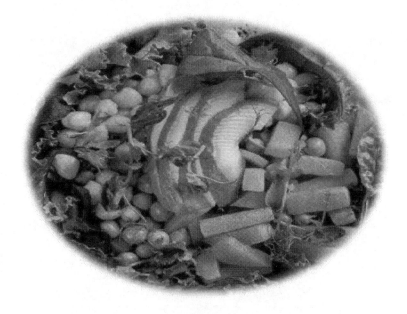

Salad Tangorana

Prep time: 10 minutes

Cook time: 35 minutes

Servings: 4-6

Ingredients:

½ cup of walnuts

2 cups of baby spinach leaves

2 oranges

1 cup of cooked quinoa

2 Teaspoons of thyme

2 Tablespoons of cold-pressed olive oil

2 sweet potatoes, peel and chopped in quarter

2 large beets, peel and chopped in quarter

Orange Dressing

2 teaspoons of honey

1 teaspoon of seeded mustard

2 Tablespoon of apple cider vinegar

Orange juice

½ cup of olive oil

Salt to taste

Pepper to taste

Preparations:

1. Heat up the oven to 350°F.

2. Coat the sweet potatoes and beets with thyme and olive oil, wrap each piece of potato and beet in foil. Cook for 35 minutes, then chop into small sizes.

3. Cook quinoa the way instructed in the package.

4. Peel the oranges and collect the juice in a jar, remove orange pith into in different parts into a bowl to get the juice.

5. Combine orange juice with the dressing ingredients including and mix properly.

6. Place the salad ingredients in a bowl and drizzle with the dressing, mix in and serve!

Ageing Resistance Salad

Prep time: 10 minutes

Servings: 2

Ingredients:

1-2 teaspoon of extra virgin olive oil

1/2 cubed avocado

3/4 cup of cherry tomatoes, divided

4 roasted and chopped parsnips

Dash salt and pepper

Preparations:

1. Wash and prepare.

2. Combine the ingredients together in a bowl and carefully mix with a spoon, to avoid mashing the ingredients.

3. Serve salad with extra garnish of salt and pepper, enjoy!

Pumpkin Seeds With Kale And Strawberry Salad

Prep time: 10 minutes

Servings: 1 serving

Ingredients:

Salad:

1/3 diced avocado, (optional)

1 tablespoon of pumpkin seeds

3 medium roasted and diced parsnips

2 sliced strawberries

2 cups of baby kale

Dressing:

Salt and pepper to taste

½ teaspoon of oregano

2-3 Tablespoon of olive oil

1 lemon Juice

Preparations:

1. Place the salad ingredients in a serving bowl.

2. Mix the dressing ingredients together in a separate small bowl.

3. Drizzle the dressing over the salad and toss to combine. Enjoy!

Guacamole Salad Thyroid-Friendly

Prep time: 10 minutes

Servings 4

Ingredients:

1 bunch of chopped fresh coriander

½ cup of pickled japalenos

2 chopped scallions

1 deseeded and chopped red pepper

1 small finely chopped red onion

2 cups of cherry tomatoes

2 chopped Lebanese cucumber

2 chopped avocados

Preparations:

1. Combine all the salad ingredient in a bowl, drizzle with extra olive oil, Season with salt and pepper and drizzle with your desired salad dressing mix in and enjoy.

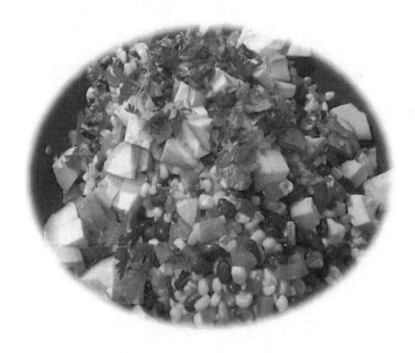

Mixed Bell Pepper, Avocado And Corn Salad

Prep time: 15-20 minutes

Servings: 6-8 servings

Ingredients:

Salad:

¼ cup chopped fresh cilantro

1 cubed avocado

1 seeded and chopped orange red bell pepper

1 seeded and chopped red bell pepper

1 ear of corn, kernels removed, boiled

1 15-oz can black beans, drain and rinse

Dressing:

Salt and pepper to taste

2 tablespoon of olive oil

1 lime juice

Preparations:

1. Place the salad ingredients in a serving bowl.

2. Mix the dressing ingredients together in a separate small bowl.

3. Drizzle the dressing over the salad and mix to combine. Enjoy!

Super Simple Salad

Prep time: 15 minutes

Servings: 2

Ingredients:

Salad:

2 tbsp slivered almonds or vegan parmesan

½ apple, sliced thin

2 (200 g) cups of thinly sliced Brussels sprouts, shaved

Dressing:

Sea salt and pepper

3 tablespoon of fresh lemon juice

¼ (60 ml) cup olive oil

Ingredients:

1. Place the Brussels into a bowl add sliced apples and toss together.

2. Mix the dressing ingredients together in a separate small bowl.

3. Drizzle the dressing over the salad and mix to combine. Enjoy!

Liver Rescue Vegetable "Bone" Broth

Prep time: 10 minutes

Cook time: 1 hour-1 hour 15 minutes

Servings: 4-6

Ingredients:

½ teaspoon of black pepper

1 teaspoon of sea salt

½ cup of fresh parsley leaves

2 teaspoons of turmeric powder

1 cup of dried shiitake mushrooms

2 4-inch kombu pieces (an edible kelp)

1 Tablespoon of apple cider vinegar or half lemon juice

6 cups of filtered water

1 cup of greens (broccoli, collards or kale)

2 carrots, chopped

2 chopped celery sticks

1 finely chopped leek

1 chopped onion

1 finely chopped knob ginger

2 finely chopped small garlic cloves

1 Tablespoon of coconut oil

Preparations:

1. Combine all the soup ingredients into a large pot, cook until heated through and then cover and simmer about 1 hour or more.

2. Strain the broth into a mason jar or large bowl. Serve warm.

Note: Can be stored in the fridge in an airtight container up to a week.

Super Green soup

Prep time: 15 minutes
Cook time: 20 minutes
Servings: 4

Ingredients:

Sea salt and pepper, to taste
1 handful of fresh basil
2 1/2 (375 ml) cups of vegetable stock
2 chopped swiss chard leaves, including stems
1 large handful of chopped spinach leaves
2 chopped large kale leaves
2 diced zucchinis
1 deseeded and chopped long green chilli
4 finely chopped garlic cloves
1 thinly sliced leek
1 Tablespoon of olive oil or coconut oil
(Optional garnish) 2 kale leaves and 4 tbsp slivered almonds or pine nuts

Preparations:

1. Warm up the oven to 350 F.
2. In a medium pot, heat the oil and sauté garlic and leek and over medium-low heat until soft.
3. Meanwhile for the optional garnish, rub oil into 2 kale leaves, lightly season with salt then line a baking tray. Bake in the preheated oven until crispy, for 10-15 mins. When it's about 6 minutes to the end, add the nuts to toast lightly.
4. Add the basil, leafy greens and zucchini into the sauté leek and garlic, stir for a few minutes.
5. Pour in the vegetable stock, cook until heated through then simmer on low heat for 5 to 8 minutes or until vegetables are tender.
6. Pour Soup into a blender and blend until smooth or blend soup using a stick blender for a smooth texture.
7. Garnish with the toasted nuts and crispy kale. Enjoy!

Sweet Potato & Kale Chili

Prep time: 10 minutes

Cook time: 25 minutes

Total time: 35 minutes

Servings: 4

Ingredients:

1 (70g) cup of chopped kale

½ tsp of salt

1/4 tsp of paprika

1/4 tsp of chili powder

1/2 tsp of cumin

1 cup of vegetable broth

1 (250g) medium peeled sweet potato, diced into small cubes

2 chopped Portobello mushrooms

1 (425g) 14.5oz can of diced tomatoes

3 chopped cloves garlic

1 chopped onion

1 tbsp of coconut oil or olive oil

Optional garnishing: avocado or slices fresh cilantro for garnish

Preparations:

1. Cook coconut oil, garlic and onion over medium heat in a pot for 2 minutes.

2. Add in the remaining ingredients with the exception of kale. Simmer with the lid on over low- medium heat, stirring occasionally about 25 minutes or until potatoes are tender.

3. Stir in chopped kale, stirring until kale is wilted. Serve and enjoy.

SOUP RECIPES

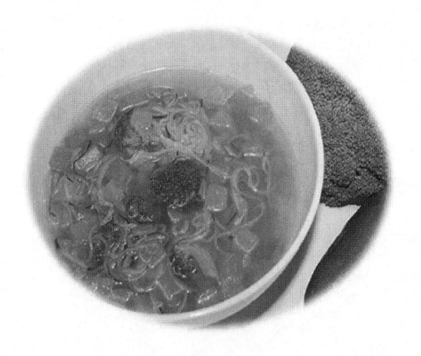

Creamy Soup

Prep time: 30 minutes
Cook time: 1 hour, 30 minutes
Servings: 6

Ingredients:

4 cups vegetable stock concentrate
3 crushed garlic cloves
2 (400g) peel and chopped medium potatoes
2 trimmed leeks, halved lengthways and sliced thinly
2 tablespoon of coconut oil
4 (600g) medium beets, trimmed
Sea salt and pepper, to taste

Preparations:

1. Warm up the oven to 350 F.
2. Wrap each beets in foil and bake in the preheated oven until soft for 50-60 minutes.
3. Remove the roasted beets from the foil then peel and chop. Try putting on a gloves so your hands won't become red.
4. Over medium heat, pour oil in saucepan and sauté garlic, potatoes and leeks, about 5 minutes or until leeks are tender. Add pepper, vegetable stock and beets.
6. Cook with the lid on until heated through, then simmer for 20 minutes.
7. Pour Soup into a blender and blend until smooth or blend soup using a stick blender for a smooth texture. Season with salt and pepper. Add some coconut cream, or chives.

Butternut Squash Creamy Soup

Prep time: 20 minutes
Cook time: 15 minutes
Servings: 4 to 6

Ingredients:

1 bay leaf
3 cups of vegetable broth
2 carrots, chopped
1/3 peeled butternut squash, seeded and coarsely chopped
½ cauliflower head, chopped coarsely

2 crushed garlic cloves
1 inch of fresh grated turmeric
1 chopped yellow onion
1 tablespoon of coconut or olive oil
1 cup unsalted raw cashews
Salt and pepper to taste

Preparations:

1. Add cashews in a spice blender or a high speed blender to grind into a coarse flour.
2. Heat the coconut or olive oil in a soup pot. Over medium heat, sauté the turmeric, onion, and garlic until onions are soft.
3. Add in the carrots, cauliflower and butternut squash, stirring for a few minutes.
5. Add in the bay leaf, vegetable stock and cashew meal, then bring to a boil.
6. Reduce to low heat and simmer until the vegetables are tender, about 15 minutes.
7. Pour Soup into a blender and blend until smooth or blend soup using a stick blender for a smooth texture. Season with pepper and salt to taste.

Coconut, Pumpkin-Cauli- Soup

Prep time: 20 minutes
Cook time: 25 minutes
Servings: 6

Ingredients:

2 (500 ml) cups of vegetable broth or stock
1 (250 ml) cup of coconut milk
½ pumpkin (500 g), coarsely chopped
½ (350 g) cauliflower head, coarsely chopped
3 crushed garlic cloves
1 (2.5 cm) fresh grated turmeric grated or 1 teaspoon dried
1 sliced leek
1 tablespoon of olive or coconut oil
Salt and pepper, to taste

Preparations:

1. Heat the coconut or olive oil in a soup pot. Over medium heat, sauté the turmeric, leek, and garlic until soft.

2. Add in the cauliflower and pumpkin, stirring for few minutes.

3. Pour in coconut milk, stirring for a minute then add the vegetable broth or stock and season with Salt and pepper to taste.

4. Cook until heated through then simmer on low heat until the vegetables are soft, about 15 minutes.

5. Pour Soup into a blender and blend until smooth or blend soup using a stick blender for a smooth texture. You can also chop vegetables into small pieces and add.

6. Add coconut milk and enjoy immediately.

Nutritious Green Soup

Prep time: 20 minutes
Cook time: 15 minutes
Servings: 6

Ingredients:

1 teaspoon of dried tarragon
1 teaspoon of dried oregano
Salt and pepper, to taste
1 handful of fresh parsley
3 (750 ml) cups of vegetable broth or stock
500 g of fresh or frozen baby peas
1 chopped zucchini
4 chopped kale leaves
1/2 chopped head of broccoli
3 crushed garlic cloves
1 sliced leek
1 tablespoon of olive oil

Preparations:

1. Heat the coconut or olive oil in a soup pot. Over medium heat, sauté the leek and garlic until soft.

2. Add in the zucchini, kale and broccoli, and stirring for few minutes.

3. Add the vegetable broth or stock and peas and cook until heated through then rest ingredients and simmer on low heat until the vegetables are soft, about 10 minutes.

4. Pour Soup into a blender and blend until smooth or blend soup using a stick blender for a smooth texture. You can also chop vegetables into small pieces and add

5. (Optional) garnish with fresh herbs and serve immediately.

Vegetable Zucchinis Soup

Prep time: 20 minutes
Cook time: 20 minutes
Servings: 4

Ingredients:

2 zucchinis
1 bay leaf
Black pepper, to taste
Sea salt to taste
6 (1.5 L) cups of vegetable stock or broth
½ chop stem and broccoli head, and florets
¼ chopped butternut squash
2 chopped carrots
(Optional) 1 teaspoon of dried turmeric
2 chopped celery stalks
1 (2.5 cm) grated ginger
3 crushed garlic cloves
1 chopped large brown onion
1 tablespoon of olive oil

Preparations:

1. Heat the coconut or olive oil in a soup pot. Over medium heat, sauté the celery, ginger and garlic until soft
2. Add in the butternut squash, carrots and turmeric and stirring for a few minutes.
3. Add the rest soup ingredients with the exception of zucchini, and cook until heated through then simmer on low heat for 10 to 15 minutes or until the vegetables are tender.
4. Cut the zucchini into fine noodles using a mandolin or spiralizer then chop long ways.
5. Pour the Soup into the soup, mix and serve immediately.

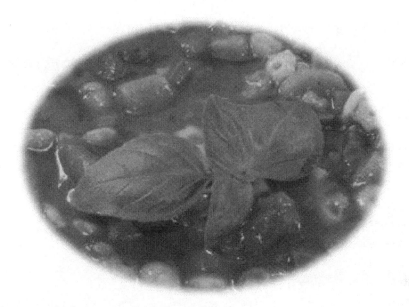

Ginger Broccoli And Spinach Soup

Prep time: 10 mins
Cook time: 25 mins
Serving: 4

Ingredients:

1/4 tsp of Black pepper
4 cup of chopped Broccoli
2 medium chopped Celery stalk
1 tablespoon of extra virgin olive oil
2 chopped Garlic cloves
1 tablespoon of minced Ginger root
2 teaspoon of Lemon juice to taste
1/2 cup of roughly chopped fresh Parsley
3 parsnips peeled, cored, chopped
1/4 teaspoon of Sea salt to taste
7 cup of Spinach
4 cup of Water

Preparations:

1. Heat olive oil in a large pot over medium heat and stir in the onion, ginger and garlic. Add the parsley, celery, parsnips, spinach and broccoli and stir briefly until the spinach is wilted.

2. Add the necessary measure of water needed to cover the vegetables at first. You can add more water to thin the soup out later.

3. Simmer on high, cover and simmer on medium heat, about 15 minutes or until the veggies are tender.

4. Puree the soup with an immersion blender add a squeeze of citrus.

Creamy Red Lentil And Kale Soup

Prep time: 5 mins

Cook time: 50 mins

Serving: 6

Ingredients:

1/2 medium diced Yellow onion

2 3/4 cup of Vegetable stock

2 tablespoons of canned tomato sauce

1 teaspoon of Sea salt

3 diced Roma tomatoes Kale

1 1/2 cup of Red lentils, raw

1 cup of chopped Kale

1 1/2 teaspoon of Cumin

1 (13.5 oz) can of Coconut milk

1/4 teaspoon of Cayenne pepper

Preparations:

1. Combine all ingredients, reserving the coconut milk and chopped kale into a medium pot, stir and cook until heated through.

2. Reduce heat to medium-low and simmer with the lid on, stirring occasionally for 30 - 40 minutes or until the lentils are tender.

3. Turn heat off heat, add coconut milk and chopped kale, stir well. Adjust salt, if needed. Enjoy!

⍰

Liver Healthy Healing Soup

Prep time: 15 mins
Cook time: 25 mins
Serving: 4

Ingredients:

1 tablespoon of coconut oil
200ml, magnesium-free, yeast-free vegetable stock
1 brown onion, roughly chopped
4 garlic cloves, roughly chopped
1 handful of roughly chopped cashews
2 tablespoon of chopped dill
1 red bell pepper, roughly chopped and deseeded
2 carrots, chopped
1 large handful of spinach
1 large sweet potato, chopped
1 avocado
1 can (200g) lentils (drained and washed)

Preparations:

1. Heat coconut oil in a large saucepan, and sauté the garlic and onion. Add carrots, and sweet potato into the pan, stir to combine, about 2 minutes.
2. Add in vegetable stock, and simmer until the vegetables are just soft but not overcooked, about 10 minutes. Add the lentils, simmer for 5 minutes.
3. If you don't have a big blender, you will have to do this in batches. Transfer into a blender and add in the dill, spinach, capsicum, and avocado. Reserve a few sprigs of dill back for garnish.
4. Puree until smooth. Serve with sprigs of dill, sprinkle with the cashews.

Justified Broccoli-Creamy Avocado Soup

Prep time: 10 mins
Cook time: 15 mins
Servings: 4

Ingredients:

Some fresh cilantro, basil, cumin to taste
Celtic Sea Salt to taste
2 cups of yeast-free vegetable broth
1 celery stalk
1 green or red pepper
1 chopped yellow onion
1 small avocado
2-3 chopped broccoli flowers

Preparations:

1. Warm up the vegetable broth (do not cook).
2. Add chopped broccoli and onion, and heat until broccoli is soft.
3. Transfer into the blender, add the celery, pepper and avocado, and puree until you have a creamy soup is creamy (add water if too thick).

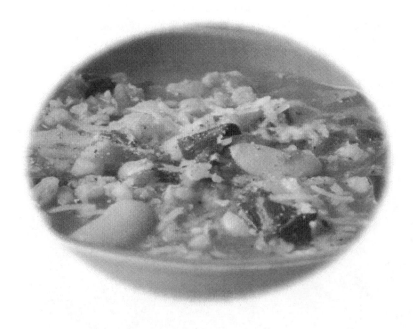

Cauliflower Soup

Prep time: 10 mins
Cook time: 10 mins
Servings: 2

Ingredients:

2 cups of cauliflower pieces
1 cup of potatoes, cut in cubes
2 cups of yeast-free vegetables stock
3 tablespoon of Swiss Emmenthal cheese, cut in cubes
2 tablespoon of fresh chives
1 tablespoon of pumpkin seeds
1 pinch of cayenne pepper and nutmeg
Salt and pepper (optional)

Preparations:

1. Warm vegetable stock in a soup pot and cook the potato and cauliflower for 5-6 minutes or until soft, and then puree with a blender.
2. Season with and cayenne pepper and nutmeg, and salt and pepper (optional).
3. Add fresh chives and emmenthal cheese and stir for some minutes until the soup is smooth. Garnish with pumpkin seeds.

Friendly Meatless Soup

Prep time: 15 mins
Cook time 40 mins
Servings: 4-6

Ingredients:

1/4 cup of your preferred pasta
2 minced garlic cloves
28 ounce can of diced plum tomatoes
1/8 tsp black pepper, freshly ground
1/4 tsp of salt
1/4 tsp of dried oregano
2 tbsp basil, finely chopped or 1 tsp of dried basil
3/4 cup of diced celery
1 cup of cannellini beans

1 cup of carrots, peeled and sliced

2 cups of diced zucchini

3 cups of water

3/4 cup of chopped onion

1 tbsp of extra virgin olive oil

Preparations:

1. Heat-up a broad saucepan over medium heat.

2. Add oil and sauté the onion, about 4 minutes, stirring not too often, until browned a bit.

3. With the exception of pasta, add in the rest ingredients and bring to a boil.

4. Reduce to low heat and simmer with the lid on for 25 minutes, stirring occasionally.

5. Add and cook pasta according to package instructions, about 10-12 minutes until pasta is al dente.

⬚

Best Liver Healing Mushroom Soup

Prep time: 10 mins

Cook time: 35 mins

Servings: 4

Ingredients:

2 cups of unsweetened almond or cashew milk

Black pepper, freshly ground

2 cups of organic vegetable broth

2 tablespoons of tapioca flour

1 tablespoon of liquid aminos

1 tsp salt

2 dried bay leaves

20 stalks of fresh thyme, leaves removed

2 10 oz packages of sliced baby portobello mushroom

2 (10 oz) packages of sliced white button mushroom

2 large diced white onions

Preparations:

1. Cook diced onions, about 5 to 7 minutes in a large saucepan over medium heat, cover to sweat them,

2. Gather the onions towards the sides of the saucepan, add mushrooms to the middle of the saucepan, and cook for 5 minutes without covering.
3. Mix the mushrooms and onions together, add in the thyme and keep cooking, about 10 minutes or more.
4. Add the liquid aminos, bay leaf and salt to the mushrooms.
5. Mix the vegetable broth and tapioca starch in a small bowl until no more lump and well combined. Pour the mixture into the mushrooms and stir, then add almond milk.
6. Cook about 15 minutes, stirring not too often. Adjust taste with freshly ground black pepper.
You can add Parmesan cheese, cashew cheese if desired.

☐

Arugula And Broccoli Liver Detox Soup

Prep time: 3 mins
Cook time 20 mins
Servings: 2

Ingredients:
1/2 lemon Juice
1 cup of arugula leaves, packed
1/4 teaspoon of dried thyme
1/4 teaspoon of freshly ground black pepper
1/4 teaspoon of salt
2 1/2 cups of water
1 (about 2/3 pound) head broccoli, cut into little florets,
1/2 yellow or Spanish onion, roughly diced
1 clove of garlic, chopped
1 tablespoon olive oil

Preparations:
1. Heat oil over medium in a large saucepan, Cook onion in the heated oil until translucent.
2. Pour in garlic and cook for additional 60 seconds, add broccoli, and keep cooking about 4 minutes more or until it is bright green. Add pepper, salt, thyme and water.
Allow to heat through, then lower heat and cook with the lid on, around 8 minutes or until broccoli is tender.

3. Blend the soup in a blender or use an immersion blender, add arugula, blend until smooth. Serve with lemon juice.

Unique Healthy Soup with Kale

Prep time: 10 mins

Cook time 1 hour 10 mins

Servings:

Ingredients:

2 cups of kale, chopped

¼ cup of steel cut oats or barley

¼ cup of lentils. Any will do

¼ cup of wild rice

¼ cup of French lentils

4 cups of vegetarian broth

Preparations:

1. Cook the broth until heated through and add other ingredients, stir.
2. Simmer on low with the lid on for 45 minutes to 1 hour.
3. Add kale, stir and simmer for 10 more minutes. Serve and enjoy.

Garnished Pear Soup Red

Prep time: 10 mins

Cook time 40 mins

Servings: 7

Ingredients:

1/2 tsp of ground black pepper

1/2 tsp of dried crushed red pepper

1 (32-oz.) container of no-fat chicken broth

2 peeled and sliced Anjou pears

Pinch of ground red pepper

2 sliced shallots

2 sliced carrots

3 large sliced red bell peppers

2 tsp of olive oil

2 tbsp of butter

1/4 tsp of salt

Garnishes: fresh pears (thinly sliced), chopped fresh chives, plain yogurt (optional)

Preparations:

1. Melt oil with butter over medium heat in a Dutch oven; add bell pepper, shallots
Carrots and Anjou pears, and sauté until tender, about 8 to 10 minutes.
2. Stir in chicken broth and ground black pepper, red pepper, ground red pepper, and salt. Cook until heated through; cover, and simmer on low heat for 25 to 30 minutes. Allow cooling 20 minutes.
3. In a food processor, Process soup, in batches until smooth, scraping the sides down as necessary. Transfer back to Dutch oven to keep warm until you are ready to use. Garnish, if desired.

[?]

LUNCH RECIPES

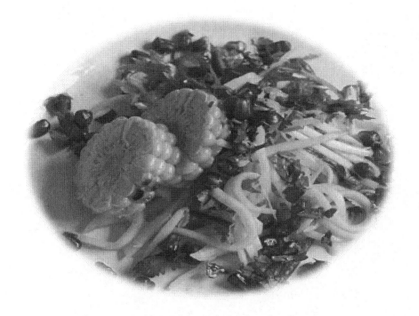

Hemp Seeds With Spicy Steamed Greens

Prep time: 10 minutes

Cook time: 5 minutes

Servings: 2-4 servings

Ingredients:

(Optional) 1 fresh chopped chili

¼ cup of hemps seeds

2 cloves garlic

1 Tablespoon of tamari

1 large thickly sliced zucchini

1 chopped broccoli

Salt and black pepper to taste

1 large asparagus bunch, ends discard and chopped in half

Preparations:

1. Lightly Steam the greens for a few minutes. (Avoid over overcooking)

2. Arrange the steamed greens on a serving dish and season with the remaining ingredients. Serve and enjoy!

Healthy Roasted Brussels Sprouts & Vinaigrette

Prep time: 20 minutes

Cook time: 25 minutes

Servings: 6

Ingredients:

4 tablespoon of dried cranberries

Sea salt and pepper, to taste

2 tablespoon of extra virgin olive oil

2 cups (200 g) Brussels sprouts, end removed and chopped in half

1 small peeled butternut squash, seeded and Cut into ½ inch chunks

Vinaigrette

Sea salt and pepper, to taste

3 tablespoon of extra virgin olive oil

2 tablespoon of rice wine vinegar

3 teaspoon of Dijon mustard

Preparations:

1. Warm up the oven to 450 F.

2. Line foil on a large baking sheet, place the veggies and drizzle with olive oil, then toss to coat. Add salt and pepper.

3. Place in the preheated oven and roast for half an hour, tossing halfway through.

4. Towards the final minutes of baking, add the cranberries.

5. Meanwhile, Combine all Vinaigrette ingredients in a blender and blend until you have smooth mixture

6. When the veggies are roasted, remove from oven and allow cooling for 5 minutes.

7. Add Dijon vinaigrette then toss to evenly coat. Serve warm and enjoy!

Easy Veggie Hash

Prep time: 10 minutes

Cook time: 25 minutes

Servings: 4

Ingredients:

1 tbls of fresh parsley, chopped

Red pepper flakes

Salt and pepper

2 cups of Swiss chard, chopped coarsely

15-oz can of black beans, drain and rinse

1 diced medium sweet potato

2 diced red potatoes

1 tbls of fresh sage leaves

3 minced cloves garlic or more

1 diced red bell pepper

1 large diced onion

3 tablespoons of olive oil

Preparations:

1. Heat the oil in a broad skillet over high-medium heat.

2. Add in onion, sage, garlic, pepper, sweet potato and red potato, cook stirring not too often, about 15 to 20 minutes or until the potatoes are soft.

2. Add in Swiss chard and beans, cook and stir for about 3 minutes until the chard wilts. Season with red pepper flakes, pepper and salt. Garnish with chopped parsley.

Pleased Stuffy Sweet Potatoes

Prep time: 15 minutes
Cook time: 1 hour
Servings: 2

Ingredients:

Fresh ground black pepper to taste
½ teaspoon of chipotle powder
½ teaspoon of cumin
¼ cup of salsa
½ diced tomato
½ diced avocado
2 large chopped kale leaves
1 tablespoon of chopped scallions
1 minced garlic clove
½ red onion, diced
½ diced red pepper
Sea salt to taste
½ cup of black beans, (BPA free canned or cooked from dried, fist soak overnight, then drain and rinse before cooking)
1 medium sweet potato

Preparations:

1. Warm up the oven to 450 F.
2. Wash and pierce the sweet potato once or twice with a fork.
3. Bake the sweet potato in the pre-warm oven for about an hour, until the middle is soft.
4. In the meantime, prepare the veggies. When the potatoe is ready, slice into two and set aside in a bowl to cool a bit.
5. Drain and rinse if using can. Combine the beans, onion, pepper, and tomato in a bowl, season with the spices, stir with the veggies to coat.
6. Add veggie and beans mixture to the potato bowl. Garnish with salsa and scallions. Add diced avocado over the top

Hearty Meatless Pie

Prep time: 10 minutes

Cook time: 40 minutes

Servings: 6

Ingredients:

1/2 cup of non-dairy milk, unsweetened

1/4 tsp of pepper

1/2 tsp of sea salt

2 tsp of tamari

1 tsp of dried thyme

2 cups of canned black-eyed peas, rinsed well and drained

2 cups of fresh trimmed green beans, cut into 1-inch sizes

4 tbsp of olive oil

2 minced cloves garlic

2 large chopped yellow onions

5 carrots, chopped

3 large peeled and chopped sweet potatoes

Preparations:

1. Warm up the oven to 400 F.

2. Pour 4 quarts of water in a large pot, bring to a boil and add the sweet potatoes, cook until fork tender for about 10 minutes.

3. In the meantime, add olive oil in a broad skillet, sauté the garlic, onions and carrots in skillet, about 5 minutes.

4. When carrot is a bit soft, add the green beans, cooking for 5 more minutes. Pour the tamari, peas, salt, thyme, and pepper. Stir altogether.

5. Transfer the mixture to a broad 10-cup baking dish.

6. Drain the potatoes and mash with half cup of non-dairy milk. Add the mashed potatoes to the top of the filling.

7. Place in the oven and bake for 30 minutes.

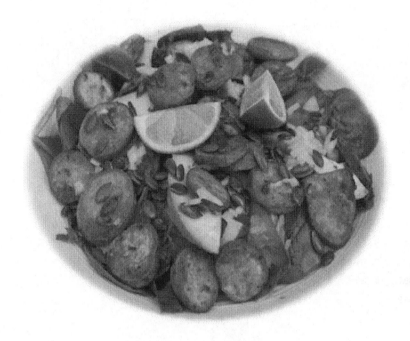

Creamy Mushroom Omelet

Prep time: 3 mins
Cook time 5 mins
Servings: 1

Ingredients:

¼ cup of chopped kale
¼ cup of diced tomato
1 tsp of minced garlic
¼ cup of chopped green onion
1 tbsp of low fat sour cream or heavy cream
2 eggs
Optional additions:
1 scoop of Daily Turmeric Tonic
¼ cup of diced mushroom
1/8 cup of diced Serrano pepper
¼ cup of chopped bell pepper

Preparations:

1. Beat sour cream and eggs together in a bowl until fluffy.
2. Sauté the onion, kale, tomato and garlic for 2-3 minutes in a small non-stick pan over medium heat until soft, add optional ingredients if using.
3. Add beaten eggs and cook for 3 minutes.
4. Flip and cook omelet for 60 seconds more.
5. Fold omelet into half and cook more about half minutes on each side.

⁈

Oven Baked Black Bean Brownies

Prep time: 20 mins
Cook time 18 mins
Servings 9-12

Ingredients:

1/2 cup of chocolate chips
1/2 tsp of baking powder
2 tsp of pure vanilla extract, alcohol-free
1/4 cup of coconut oil
1/2 cup of pure maple syrup
1/4 tsp of salt
1/2 cup of quick oats
2 tbsp of cocoa powder
1 15-oz can of organic black beans, drained and rinsed

Preparations:

1. Heat up the oven to 350 F.
2. Add every ingredients in a food processor, but reserve the chips, process until totally smooth.
3. Add the chocolate chips, stir.
4. Transfer into the oven and bake for 18 minutes.
5. Allow cooling completely out of the oven before cutting. If not satisfied with the texture, chilled in the refrigerator overnight to firm up.

⁈

Liver Pass Fresh Turmeric Rice

Prep time: 20 mins

Cook time 55 mins

Servings 4-6

Ingredients:

2 1/2 cups of vegetable stock or water

2 grated cloves garlic

1 tsp of grated fresh turmeric or 1/4 tsp of ground turmeric

1/4 cup of golden raisins

1 cup of brown rice (short-grain)

1/2 cup of onions, diced

2 tsps of coconut oil

Pinch of Salt

Pinch of pepper

Preparations:

1. Heat coconut oil the saucepan over medium heat, pour the onions and sauté, about 4 minutes until soft and translucent.

2. Add in the raisins, rice, garlic and turmeric. Stir.

3. Sauté about 2 minutes or until you perceive the aroma, add the stock.

4. Bring to a boil, then cook on low heat, about 45 minutes with the lid on or until rice is tender.

5. Turn the heat off, still leaving lid on for 5 minutes to steam the rice.

6. Uncover and add the season, fluff with a fork before serving.

Mushrooms Oregano toasted wheat rolls

Prep time: 5 mins

Cook time 15 mins

Servings: 4

Ingredients:

4 split and toasted, whole-wheat rolls

3 Oz of reduced-fat provolone cheese, thinly sliced

1 tbsp of reduced-sodium soy sauce

1/4 cup of vegetable broth

1 tbsp of all-purpose flour

1/2 tsp of freshly ground pepper

2 tsp of dried oregano

1 large red bell pepper, thinly sliced

4 large sliced Portobello mushrooms, gills and stems removed

1 sliced medium onion

2 tsp of extra-virgin olive oil

Preparations:

1. In a Broad nonstick pan over medium-high heat, heat olive oil, add onion, cook ,about 5 minutes stirring frequently, until tender and starting to brown.

2. Add oregano, pepper, mushrooms and bell pepper, cook, about 7 minutes, stirring frequently, until the vegetables are tender.

3. Lower heat and sprinkle flour on the vegetables, stir to coat. Stir in soy sauce and broth; bring to a simmer.

4. Turn off heat, place slices of the cheese on the vegetables, cover with a lid and let stand, 1 to 2 minutes until cheese melts.

5. Spoon mixture with a spatula into 4 parts, keeping the melted cheese layer on top. Serve immediately by Spooning a portion of the mixture onto each toasted bun.

?

Special Turkey With Veggie Stuffed Peppers

Prep time: 15 mins

Cook time 20 mins

Servings: 4

Ingredients:

1/2 tsp of garlic powder

1 tsp of Italian seasoning

1 tbsp of tomato paste

1 (14.5 Oz) can of diced tomatoes, drained

1 cup of fresh spinach

1/2 diced yellow bell pepper

1/2 dice green bell pepper

1 chopped zucchini

1 cup of sliced mushrooms

1/2 minced onion

2 tbsp of olive oil

1 lbs of 93 percent lean ground turkey

4 red bell peppers

Salt and pepper

Preparations:

1. Pour water into a large pot and bring to boil. Remove the seeds of the peppers and cook peppers for 5 minutes in pot; drain and set aside.

2. Heat up the oven to 350 F.

3. Cook the turkey over medium heat in a skillet, until brown evenly. Set aside.

4. Heat olive oil in the same skillet, add the spinach, yellow bell pepper, green bell pepper zucchini, and mushrooms, and onion, cook until soft.

5. Transfer turkey back to the pan, add in the rest ingredients. Add enough peppers to the mixture.

6. Arrange the peppers toward a side of casserole dish.

7. Place in the preheated oven and bake for 15 minutes.

Spinach Zucchini With Pesto

Prep time: 8 mins
Cook time: 5 mins
Serving: 4

Ingredients:

1/2 cup of cherry tomatoes sliced in half
1/2 cup of extra virgin olive oil
1/4 cup of cashews
1 small to medium lemon Juice
3 minced garlic cloves
1/4 cup of basil
3 cups of baby spinach
4 zucchinis, spiralized
Salt and Pepper to taste

Preparations:

1. Pulse cashews, garlic, basil, and spinach in a food processor until chopped finely. Then slowly add lemon juice and olive oil with food processor still running. Season with salt and pepper.

2. Combine the spinach Lemon Pesto and zucchini pasta in a serving bowl. Garnish with sliced cherry tomatoes.

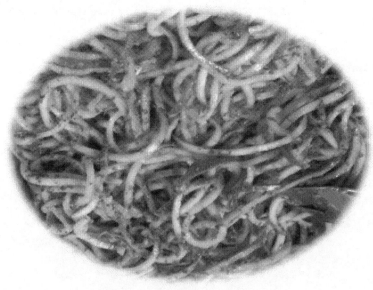

Papaya- Avocado Salad

Prep time: 10 mins
Cook time: 10 mins
Serving: 4

Ingredients:

1 cup of coarsely chopped Arugula
2 (1 cup) of small diced avocado
1/3 cup of chopped unsalted raw Cashew nuts
1/4 cup of coriander Cilantro chopped coarsely or fresh mint
3 tablespoon of fresh Lime juice
4 medium ripe Papaya, divided
2 chopped small shallot
1 finely chopped medium Yellow onion

Preparations:

1. Slice 2 papayas and remove the seeds. Set aside.
2. Peel the other 2 papayas using a vegetable peeler, slice into two and remove the seeds. Dice the peeled and seeded papaya into half-inch sizes, set aside in a bowl.
3. Add shallots, lime juice, cilantro, cashews, and avocados to the peeled and diced papayas, toss together to combine. Season with pepper and salt. Carefully mix in arugula. Serve salad in the papaya halves.

Easy Healthy Risotto

Prep time: 15 mins
Cook time: 35 mins
Serving: 4

Ingredients:

1 handful of parsley, chopped
1 can of garbanzo beans, rinse thoroughly
2 tablespoons of capers
1 jar artichoke hearts, drained
1 bunch of Swiss chard, cut into ribbons
3 minced cloves garlic
Artichokes medium
1 thinly sliced shallot
2 tablespoon of coconut oil

1 cup of quinoa, rinse and drained

2 cups of yeast free vegetable broth

Salt and pepper (Himalayan, Celtic Grey, or Redmond Real Salt)

Preparations:

1. Add vegetable broth and quinoa in a pot and cook the quinoa over high heat.

2. Cover and reduce heat to low when the water comes to a boil, cook for 20 minutes or until quinoa is cooked and water is absorbed. Set aside.

3. Meanwhile, heat the coconut oil in a sauté pan, add shallots and cook, about 8 minutes until melted. Add Swiss chard and garlic, cook for 5 minutes more. Add artichokes, capers and garbanzo beans and cook for 2 minutes extra.4. Toss the Swiss chard mixture and quinoa in a bowl. Add parsley garnish and season with pepper and sea salt.

🄯

Unique Quinoa Stuffed Squash

Prep time: 60 mins

Cook time: 55 mins

Serves: 2

Ingredients:

1 teaspoon of garlic powder

2 teaspoon of dried thyme

1 1/2 cup of cooked quinoa

Black pepper to taste

1/4 cup of chopped walnuts

2 sliced spring onions, white part

1 red bell pepper, finely chopped

1 medium finely chopped shallot

1 cup of steamed green peas

2 tablespoon of coconut oil

1 big spaghetti squashes, wash and slice in half and seeded

Pink salt to taste

Preparations:

1. Heat up the oven to 400ºF

2. Bake spaghetti squashes, about 40 minutes until tender.

3. Meanwhile heat 1 tablespoon of coconut oil in a skillet and cook the bell pepper and shallot until soft. Add green peas and spices, walnuts and quinoa until heated through. Season with pepper and pink salt.
3. Fill the squash with quinoa walnuts mixture and heat in the oven for 5 – 8 minutes. Serve with fresh greens.

Roasted Cauliflower And Coriander

Prep time: 15 mins
Cook time: 15 mins
Serving: 4

Ingredients:
1 tablespoon chopped roughly mint
2 tablespoons of chopped roughly coriander/cilantro
1/4 cup of pine nuts
1 large cauliflower, cut into bite size florets
2 teaspoons of ground turmeric (I use organic)
1 tablespoon of ground cumin
Himalayan salt to taste
1/2 cup of coconut oil

Preparations:
1. Heat up the oven to 425F
2. Combine the turmeric, coconut oil, 1/2 teaspoon of salt and cumin in a large bowl, and mix using your hands combine and warm the oil.
3. Add in the cauliflower florets, mix well to coat.
4. Pour the cauliflower on a baking tray, then spread out.
5. Transfer to the pre-warmed oven and roast until the cauliflower is tender and starting to brown, around 15-20 minutes.
6. Meanwhile chuck the pine nuts and slightly toast it on a baking tray in the oven, about a minute.
7. Serve cauliflower in a large bowl and sprinkle with the mint, coriander/cilantro and pine nuts.

⁇

DINNER RECIPES

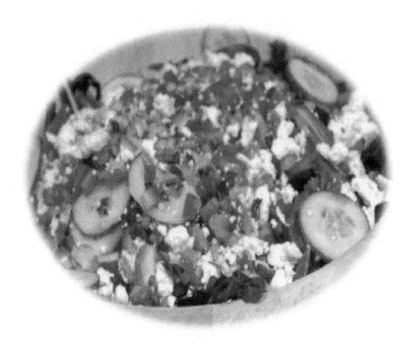

Quick Greens And Beans

Prep time: 10 minutes
Cook time: 10 minutes
Servings: 2, 4 as a snack

Ingredients:

Pinch of crushed red pepper flakes
1 tsp of cumin
14-oz can of white beans, drained and rinsed
4 cups of fresh spinach, rinse and drain
Black pepper to taste
2 minced cloves garlic
1 tbsp of olive oil
Sea salt to taste

Preparations:

1. Heat olive oil and garlic in a broad skillet, over high-medium heat.
2. Add the remaining ingredients to the skillet. Stirring frequently until the beans is cooked through and the spinach fully wilts, about 5 minutes. Season with salt and black pepper.

Seasoned Cauliflower Rice With Beans

Prep time: 15 minutes
Cook time: 10 minutes
Servings: 4

Ingredients:

2 tablespoon of your favorite hot sauce
¼ chopped chives
Fresh black pepper, to taste
Sea salt to taste
Pinch of cayenne pepper
1 tablespoon of chili powder
2 tablespoon of cumin
½ jalapeno
1 chopped garlic clove
½ red onion

1 avocado

2 tomatoes

2 (400 g) cups of black beans (BPA free canned or cooked from dried, fist soak overnight, then drain and rinse before cooking)

½ head of cauliflower, stem removed and chopped into florets

Preparations:

1. Drain and rinse. If using canned beans

2. Steam cauliflower florets with chopped garlic for about 8 minutes, until soften a bit yet firm.

3. Drain cauliflower then add in the food processor, to pulse briefly to look like rice shape.

4. Pour into a bowl and mix in hot sauce, jalapeno, tomato, onion, spices, and beans.

5. Garnish with diced avocado and chopped chives.

Liver Friendly Pesto Pasta Salad

Prep time: 10 minutes

Cook time: 10 minutes

Servings: 4

Ingredients:

Salad

4 tablespoon of chopped walnuts

4 tablespoon of currants

1/2 cup (100 g) black beans (cooked or BPA free canned)

1/2 sliced red onion

4 tablespoon of sun dried tomatoes

2 handfuls of baby spinach leaves

1 (150 g) cup of cherry tomatoes, divided

Pasta

2 – 3 large zucchini

Pesto

Sea salt and pepper, to taste

1-2 fresh crushed garlic cloves

1-2 tablespoon of lemon juice

60 – 125 ml (1/4 – 1/2) cup of extra-virgin olive oil

1/2 (70 g) cup of pine nuts

1 huge handful of firmly packed basil leaves

Preparations:

1. Use a mandolin or vegetable spiralizer, to form zucchini curls or slice thinly into thin strips.

2. Blend the pesto ingredients in a high speed blender until a smooth.

3. Lightly sauté the zucchini, then toss with the pesto and salad ingredients. Serve immediately.

Simple Steps Quinoa Salad

Prep time: 15 minutes

Cook time: 5 minutes

Servings: 4

Ingredients:

Himalayan salt, to taste

2 tablespoon of balsamic vinegar

1 tablespoon of extra virgin olive oil

1/2 (60 g) cup of chopped walnuts,

1 diced cucumber

3 small chopped orange, yellow and green bell peppers, you can use one color if you wish.

1 (250 g) cup of quinoa

Preparations:

1. Rinse and add the quinoa into a pot, fill the pot with 2 cups of water and bring to a boil, stirring regularly for about 15 minutes until water is absolved and quinoa is fluffy.

2. Prepare the peppers and cucumbers, then add cucumbers, peppers, Chop walnuts and cooked quinoa into a bowl.

3. Combine balsamic, olive oil and salt, in a separate bowl and stir.

4. Combine quinoa mixture and the dressing, mix well to combine. Cool in the fridge up to 2 hours or serve immediately.

Simple Steps Dinner Dish

Prep time: 5 minutes

Cook time: 30 minutes

Servings: 2

Ingredients:

3/4 cup of chickpeas, washed and drained, if using can

2 handfuls of spinach

1 tablespoon of olive oil

2 cups of cherry tomatoes, divided

2 chopped garlic cloves

Preparations:

1. In a sauté pan, heat oil for 2 minutes, add the chopped garlic stirring not too often until slightly browned for 2 minutes extra.

2. Add in the tomatoes, then lower to low-medium heat and cook until tomatoes are tender, about 5-10 minutes.

3. Add garbanzo beans, and cook for 5 extra minutes.

4. Add in the spinach and cook with the lid on, for 2 more minutes until the spinach is wilted. Serve and enjoy.

Dinner Style Smoothie Bowl

Prep time: 10 minutes

Servings: 2

Ingredients:

Smoothie:

2 (500 ml) cups of unsweetened almond, hemp or coconut milk

1/2 avocado

1/2 (115 g) cup of frozen raspberries or fresh raspberries

1 (225 g) cup of fresh blueberries or frozen blueberries

Toppings:

2 tablespoon of gluten free oats

Optional: Mixed of nuts, fruits and seeds

Dash of cinnamon

2 tablespoon of hemp seeds/hearts

2 tablespoon of goji berries

1/2 sliced banana

Preparations:

1 Combine all smoothie ingredients in a blender and blend for 1-2 minutes until you have smooth mixture. Pour into 2 bowls.
2. Divide toppings between smoothies bowl evenly and enjoy!

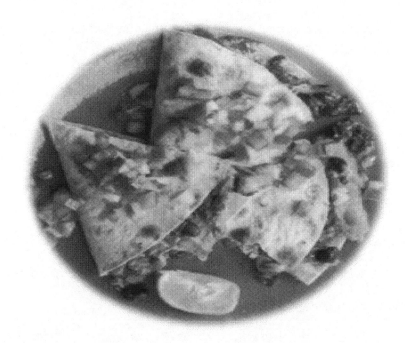

Spaghetti Squash Stuffed With Vegetable

Prep time: 5 minutes
Cook time: 20 minutes
Servings: 4 - 6

Ingredients:

1/2 teaspoon each of: herbs de Provence, oregano, basil
Salt and pepper to taste
1 lemon juice
3 handfuls of spinach
1 bunch of asparagus, cut into 1-inch pieces
6-7 peeled and chopped large carrots,
1 cup of cherry tomatoes, slice in half

2 chopped garlic cloves
1 tablespoon of olive oil
1 medium whole spaghetti squash, cut in half and seeded
Preparations:
1. Pour 1-2 inches of water in glass dish, place the spaghetti squash face down in the glass dish.
2. Heat in the microwave for 12-15 minutes on high heat or until soft or cook in the oven.
3. Meanwhile, Warm up a sauce pan over high-medium heat, add oil, carrots and garlic, cook and stir for 3-4 minutes. Add the remaining ingredients, reduce to medium-low heat and sauté until vegetables are soft and spaghetti squash is cooked.
4. When the spaghetti squash is ready, scoop the inside into the sauté pan. Mix together and add lemon juice, mix well and enjoy!
(Alternatively: You can stuff the squash with the sautéed vegetables and eat with a fork.

Chickpea Chili Quinoa with Sweet Potato
Prep time: 20 minutes
Cook time: 1 hour, 10 minutes
Servings: 6
Ingredients:
1 (230 g) cup of cooked quinoa
1/2 teaspoon of ground cumin
1/2 teaspoon of sea salt
1/2 teaspoon of dry mustard
1 tablespoon of pure maple syrup
1 tablespoon of (15 ml) honey
2 (30 g) tablespoon of chili powder
2-3 tablespoon of cinnamon
1 (250 ml) cup of apple cider or fresh apple juice plus
1 (250 ml) cup of water
2 15 ounces of BPA-free cans of chickpeas, rinse and drain
32 ounces of vegetable broth
1 BPA-free can of diced tomatoes with onion and garlic
2 (30 ml) tablespoons of olive oil

1 large diced sweet potato

Preparations:

1. Add the oil and diced potatoes in a large stockpot. Sauté about 8 minutes to until potatoes is soften.

2. Add in the rest ingredients and simmer on medium heat about 20 minutes.

3. Reduce heat to low and simmer for 40 minutes. Enjoy!

Healthy Liver Friendly Chilli Chicken

Prep time: 5 mins

Cook time 50 mins

Servings: 4

Ingredients:

Salt and pepper, to taste

1 tsps of dried chili flakes

2 tsps of grated lime zest

2 tbsp of lime juice

2 crushed cloves garlic

4 tbsp of olive oil

2 pounds of chicken drumsticks

Preparations:

1. Set chicken drumsticks aside in a bowl.

2. Combine all ingredients in a bowl and whisk thoroughly to combine, and then add the drumsticks, cover and place in the refrigerator for two hours.

3. Heat up the oven to 375 F.

4. Greased an oven tray, then transfer the chicken drumsticks on it.

5. Place in the oven and bake for about 45 minutes or until the juices run clear, flipping over just half way through the baking. Serve along with salad.

Delicious Turkey Meatloaf

Prep time: 15 mins

Cook time 1 hour

Servings: 8

Ingredients:

1 8-oz can of zero-salt-added tomato sauce
Freshly ground black pepper
1/2 tsp of salt
1/4 cup of ketchup
2 tsp of Worcestershire sauce
2 large eggs, beaten
 1/2 cup of orange or red bell pepper, seeded and chopped
2 lbs of lean ground turkey breast
1 finely chopped medium onion
1/2 cup of nonfat milk
3/4 cup of quick-cooking oats

Preparations:
1. Heat up the oven to 350°F.
2. Stir the milk and oats together in a small bowl. Leave to soak up to 3 minutes.
3. Combine every ingredients in a large bowl but reserve the tomato sauce. Stir until combined.
4. Pour the mixture into a baking dish (I use 9 x 13-inch) and form into a loaf about 2 inches high and 5 inches wide. Spread over the tomato sauce on the meatloaf.
3. Place in the preheated oven and bake until it reads 160°F when an instant-read thermometer is inserted into the meat center, about 1 hour.
4. Let rest out of the oven, about 10 to 15 minutes before slicing.

⦿

Amazing Lime Rice With Garlic Cilantro
Prep time: 5 mins
Cook time 20 mins
Servings 3

Ingredients:
Fresh cilantro, (chopped) for garnish
1 tsp of kosher salt
4 cups of low-sodium chicken broth
3 limes Juice and 2 limes zest (reserve 1 lime juice for garnish)
2 cups of long-grain rice
1 large chopped onion
3 minced cloves garlic

1 tbsp of vegetable oil

Preparations:

1. Heat the oil over medium heat in a large skillet.
2. Add onions and garlic and cook until softened, about 3 to 4 minutes.
3. Lower heat and add rice; cook, stirring constantly, about 3 minutes, making certain the rice isn't burnt.
4. Add 2 limes zest and 2 limes juice into a liquid measuring cup. Combine the lime juice and chicken broth, should give about of 4 cups.
5. Pour the juice/liquid into the rice, add salt.
6. Increase to medium heat and bring to a boil, reduce to low heat and simmer with the lid on for 10 to 15 minutes or until the rice is soft. Try and avoid the rice being sticky.
7. To serve, stir more lime juice and chopped cilantro to taste or garnish with lime wedges.

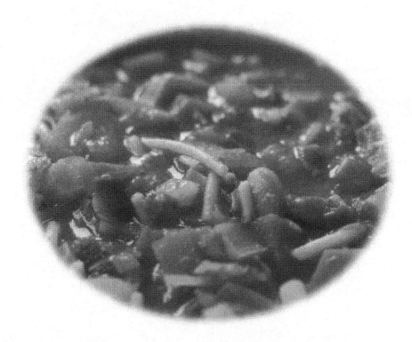

Sweet Potato, Mushrooms-Chickpea Cacciatore
Prep time 25 mins

Cook time 45 mins

Servings: 4

Ingredients:

½ cup of black olives

1 large sliced red pepper (capsicum)

3 (500g) cups of canned & drained chickpeas or cooked freshly

1/2 cup (100 g) thickly sliced button mushrooms

1 tablespoon of apple cider vinegar

1 cup (200 mls) of vegetable stock

1 tablespoon of tomato paste

14 ounces can of crushed tomatoes

1 large peeled sweet potato, chopped into bite sizes

1 large handful of finely chopped basil

1 handful of finely chopped parsley, and more for garnish

4 crushed cloves garlic

1 chopped, large brown onion

1 tablespoon of olive oil

Preparations:

1. Heat oil in a broad saucepan over medium-low heat. Add onions and garlic and sauté until the onion is tender.

2. Pour in the herbs and sauté for one minute more

3. Add the mushrooms, apple cider vinegar, tomato paste, tomatoes, vegetable stock, and sweet potato. Simmer for 10 minutes, stirring frequently.

4. Stir in the rest ingredients, simmer, stirring frequently for 10 minutes more.

5. Serve with basmati or brown rice, cauliflower rice, and garnish with parsley.

Liver Friendly Roasted Broccoli

Prep time: 5 mins

Cook time: 30 mins

Serving: 4

Ingredients:

Black pepper to taste

10 fresh garlic cloves, sliced

3 tablespoon of extra virgin olive oil

Sea salt to taste

1 large bunch broccoli florets, cut into bite size pieces

Preparations:

1. Preheat oven to 450 F.

2. Arrange the broccoli and garlic in a bowl, Add olive oil, pepper and salt. Stir well to coat

3. Spread evenly on a baking sheet and Roast about 10 minutes, then flip and roast for extra 10 to 20 minutes, or as you desired crispiness. Serve and enjoy!

Mashed parsley Cauliflower Potatoes

Prep time: 10 mins
Cook time: 15 mins
Serving: 4

Ingredients:

2 teaspoon of chopped parsley
2 teaspoon of coconut oil
1 teaspoon of garlic powder
1 carrot
1/4 cup of yeast free vegetable broth
1 chopped head of cauliflower
1 chopped onion
3 minced cloves garlic
2 teaspoon of chopped rosemary
Sea salt
Black pepper to taste

Preparations:

1. In a large pot, heat the coconut oil, sauté garlic and onion until slightly browned, about 5 minutes.
2. Add in vegetable broth, carrot, and cauliflower. Cook until heated through, then simmer for 10 minutes on medium-low. Add more of the vegetable broth if needed.
3. Add parsley, rosemary, salt, garlic powder and pepper. Mash using either an immersion blender, food processor or a blender until smooth. Enjoy!

Quinoa, white beans Sweet Potato With Carrot

Prep time: 3 mins
Cook time: 15-20 mins
Serving: 4

Ingredients:

¼ cup of extra virgin olive oil
1 lemon juice and Zest
½ cup of almond slivers
1 large bunch of sage, (cut into ribbons)
1 grated carrot

1 grated beet
1 grated sweet potato
1 15-oz can of white beans
½ bunch of Swiss chard, (cut into ribbons)
2 chopped shallots
4 minced garlic cloves
4 cups of vegetable broth
Sea salt
Black pepper
2 cups of quinoa, rinsed, soaked for 20 minutes

Preparations:

1. Cook shallots, garlic, vegetable broth, and quinoa on medium heat for 15 to 20 minutes in a pot or until liquid is absorbed. Stir in the remaining ingredients and cook until heated through. Enjoy!

⁇

DESSERT AND SNACK

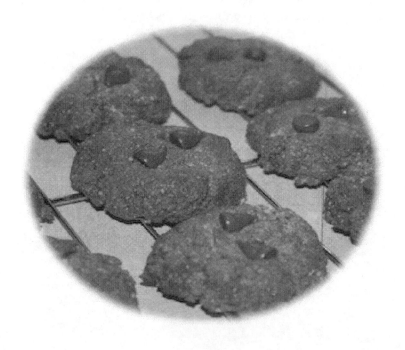

Almond- Cinnamon Porridge, Grain-Free

Prep time: 10 minutes
Cook time: 5 minutes
Servings: 2

Ingredients:

½ teaspoon of vanilla bean extract
½ teaspoon of ground cinnamon
¼ teaspoon of ground nutmeg
2 teaspoons of chia seeds
1 teaspoon of coconut oil
1/2 or less cup of almond milk
(Optional) 1 pitted date
1 chopped apple
½ cup of almonds
Pinch of salt

Preparations:

1. Chop the well nuts using a food processor.
2. Add in the apple and date, and process until well chopped and crumbly.
3. Add in the rest ingredients, mix to combine.
4. Pour into a saucepan to heat for 5 minutes over a medium heat, Cook stirring.
5. Top with a sprinkle of nutmeg, fresh chopped fruit

Smooth Sailing Muffin Crumble

Prep time: 10 minutes
Cook time: 20 minutes
Servings: 8

Ingredients:

4 tablespoon of coconut oil, slightly firm
2 tablespoon of maple syrup
1/4 (60 g) cup of buckwheat (or almonds, macadamias, chopped pecans)
2/3 (85 g) cup of chopped walnuts

2/3 (65 g) cup of almond meal

4 plums

Preparations:

1. Warm up the oven to 350F, also line a baking tray.

2. Cut the plums into two, scoop out seeds and some of the flesh to make room for the filling.

3. Mix the rest ingredients together and use your finger to rub the coconut oil in until finely combined.

4. Fill the inside of the halved plums with the mixture and place in the pre-warm oven and bake for 15 to 20 minutes or until the plums are soft. Enjoy!

Vegan Pineapple Coconut Whip

Prep time: 10 minutes

Cook time: 0 minutes

Servings: 6

Ingredients:

1/4 (60 ml) cup of coconut milk or cream

1-2 tablespoon of pure maple syrup, to taste

1/2 lime

1/2 lemon

2 (280 g) cups of frozen pineapple chunks

Preparations:

1. Combine every ingredients in a blender and blend for 1-2 minutes until you have smooth or chunky mixture as you prefer add a little fresh mint if desired. Consume immediately or chill before serve.

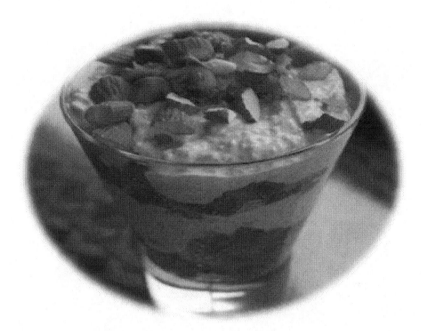

No season Apple Pie Chia Parfait

Prep time: 10 minutes

Cook time: 20 minutes

Servings: 2-4

Ingredients:

Apple pie filling

1 teaspoon of natural vanilla extract

1 teaspoon of cinnamon

2 Tablespoon of chia seeds

¾ cup of coconut water

3 large peeled apples, cored and diced

Coconut yogurt

2 Tablespoon of chopped almonds

1-2 teaspoon of maple syrup or to taste

1 teaspoon of vanilla extract

2 Tablespoon of chia seeds

2 Tablespoon of sunflower seeds

1 cup of coconut yogurt

Preparations:

1. In a bowl, combine the ingredients for coconut yogurt

2. In a saucepan, combine the ingredients for apple pie and simmer until apples are tender, about 15-20 minutes. Mash up part of the apple for a mixed consistency.

2. First Layer the apple pie filling, coconut yogurt, repeat a second time then add more apple pie filling to the top, lastly add the chopped nuts.

Healing Macadamia Cashew Peanut Butter
Prep time: 10 minutes
Servings: 30
Ingredients:
1 tablespoon of maple syrup
¼ teaspoon of sea salt
2 tablespoon of macadamia oil
1 (150 g) cup of peanuts
1 (150 g) cup of macadamia nuts, raw
1 (150 g) cup of cashews
Preparations:
1. Start by adding the nut to a blender and blend until smooth, the Combine the rest ingredients in a blender and blend for until you have smooth mixture. Can be stored up to 3 months in the fridge in an airtight container.

Seasoned Green Bean
Prep time: 5 minutes
Cook time: 5 minutes
Servings: 2
Ingredients:
 Sea salt and pepper
Chilli powder
3 (750 ml) cups of cold water
3 (750 ml) cups of hot water
2 (300 g) cups of green beans, trimmed
Preparations:

1. Bring water and a pinch of salt to a boil in a small saucepan and add green beans to blanch for a minutes or two.
2. Scoop out the beans from the saucepan and add in cold water to halt the cooking process.
3. Place the beans on a paper towel to dry then season with pepper, chilli and salt.

Cucumber With Tuna Mixture
Prep time: 15 mins
Cook time: 0 mins
Serving: 12
Ingredients:
1 can of white tuna, canned in water, drained
1 whole fresh lime juice (divided)
1 minced Garlic clove
2 teaspoon of extra virgin olive oil
1 (12 sliced) Cucumber
3 tomato Cherry Tomatoes (for garnish)
3 tomato diced Cherry Tomatoes
1 pinch of Salt and pepper
1 peeled, pitted Avocado
Preparations:
1. Mix the olive oil, drained tuna, and half lime juice together in a small bowl. Season with pepper and salt. Set aside.
2. Mash the remaining lime juice and avocado flesh with fork until partially smooth in a different small bowl. Mix in diced tomatoes and minced garlic. Season with salt and pepper.
3. Lay out cucumber slices on. Spoon small tuna mixture on each cucumber slice and cherry tomato quarter on a serving tray. Enjoy!

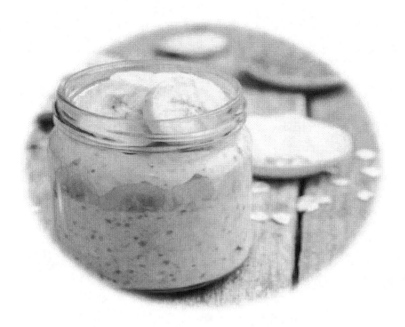

Banana Garnished Chia Seed Pudding

Prep time: 5-10 minutes

Servings: 3-4 servings

Ingredients:

1 Tablespoon of cocoa powder (optional)

Dash of cinnamon

¼ banana

½ teaspoon of vanilla

1 Tablespoon of honey

½ cup of chia seeds

2 cups of almond milk

Garnish: 1/3 banana

Preparations:

1 Combine every ingredients in a blender and blend for 1-2 minutes until you have smooth mixture

2. Transfer the mixture to serving plate and place in the refrigerator for 2 to 3 hour to set.

3. Garnish with the 1/3 banana. Enjoy!

Collard Greens Coconut vinegar Wrap

Ready time: 5

Servings: 4

Ingredients:

1 cup of Walnuts or pecans

1 thinly sliced sweet onion

1/8 teaspoon of Sea salt (to taste)

4 leaf of Collard greens

1/8 teaspoon of Coconut vinegar (to taste)

2 thinly sliced medium   Apple

Preparations:

1. Slice the leaves into two and discard the hard stem.

2. Stuff each half green with ingredients, wrap and enjoy!

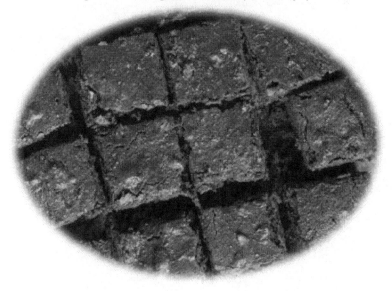

Healthy Liver Mashed Avocado Wraps

Prep time: 5 mins

Servings: 2

Ingredients:

1 organic lemon juice

1/2 bunch of chopped fresh coriander or parsley

½ fresh chopped chilli

½ medium-sized chopped red onion

3 ripe avocados

2 ripe chopped tomatoes

6 big romaine lettuce leaves,

1 pinch Himalayan crystal salt

Preparations:

1. Mash the avocados in a bowl using a fork until fine.

2. Add lemon juice and salt over the mashed avocado and mix in the parsley, coriander red onion, and tomatoes.

3. Wash the lettuce leaves and them pat dry.

4. Scoop the mixture over the lettuce leaves, wrap and keep intact with a cocktail stick!

Healthy Pumpkin Fries

Prep time: 10 mins

Cook time: 30-40 mins

Servings: 1 tray

Ingredients:

Pinch of cumin powder

½ teaspoon of cayenne pepper

1 teaspoon of organic or sea salt

¼ cup of extra virgin olive oil (cold pressed)

Pinch of curry powder

1 pumpkin

Preparations:

1. Heat up the oven to 350° F.

2. Slice pumpkin into two, discard seeds and strings, wash well and peel out the large pieces with a sharp knife. Slice the pulp just like a French Fries.

3. Lay the pumpkin slices on a tray, carefully pour in olive oil or spray with an oil sprayer, and then season with cumin powder, curry powder, pepper and salt.

4. Place in the preheated oven and bake for 30 to 40 minutes, toss occasionally.

Best Marinated Zucchini Squash

Prep time: 10 mins
Cook time: 60 mins
Serving: 4

Ingredients:

1 tablespoon of minced basil
1 tablespoon of minced dill
1 tablespoon of minced oregano
1 tablespoon of olive oil
½ cup of sun-dried tomatoes, chopped
2 fresh yellow squash
2 fresh zucchini, slice and squash thin into half mooned shape sizes
1 teaspoon of sea salt

Preparations:

1. Place the zucchini in a bowl and add the remaining ingredients, toss and allow the vegetables marinate for 30 minutes to 1 hour or steam or sauté for 4 minutes or grill for few minute

American Spicy Stewed Apples

Prep time: 15 mins
Cook time 30 mins
Servings: 4

Ingredients:

1 teaspoon of maple syrup or honey (if desired)
¼ cup of water
¼ teaspoon of ground ginger or more
1 teaspoon of ground cinnamon or more

4 apples, remove core and chopped
½ teaspoon of ground nutmeg
Preparations:
1. Pour every ingredients in a pot and heat until it simmers.
2. Reduce to low heat, stir and cook about 30 minutes, or until apples are tender.
3. Stir frequently and add water in case the mixture becomes too dry.
4. To serve dollop canned coconut cream.

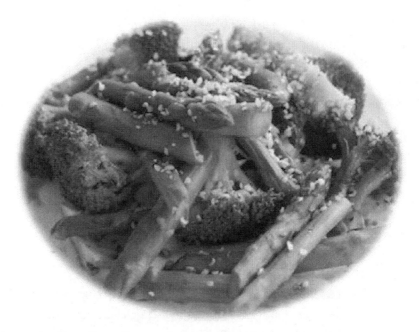

Granola Oats Bars Dessert
Prep time: 5 mins
Cook time 1 hour
Servings: 6
Ingredients:
1 1/2 cups of quick cooking rolled oats
3/4 cup of peanut butter (homemade)
1/4 cup of sliced almonds
1/4 cup of cacao nibs
2 tablespoons of honey or maple syrup
2 tablespoons of roasted flax seeds

1 tablespoon of coconut oil
1/4 teaspoon of vanilla essence
Pinch of salt
Preparations:
1. In a deep bowl, mix all ingredients together until finely combine.
2. Line butter paper on a tray, pour in the mixture and press out using your spoon or palm to form a square.
3. Place in the Refrigerator not less than an hour.
4. Cut into a rectangular of 6 equal bars.
5. Store in the refrigerator in an air-tight container.

Gifted Plum Muffin Crumble
Prep time 10 mins
Cook time 20 min
Servings 8
Ingredients:
2/3 (85 g) cup of chopped walnuts
4 tablespoons of coconut oil, slightly hardened
2 tablespoons of maple syrup
1/4 (60 g) cup of buckwheat or chopped pecans, or almonds
2/3(65 g) cup of almond meal
Plums, slice in half and remove seed
Preparations:
1. Heat up the oven to 350F and prepare a baking tray by lining it with parchment paper.
2. Scoop out some of the plum flesh into a bowl.
3. Add rest ingredients and use your fingers to rub in the coconut oil until well combined.
3. Add the mixture over the plums to and bake in the preheated oven until the plums are tender, about 15 to 20 minutes.

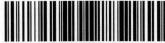

Made in the USA
Lexington, KY
11 March 2019